$7.65 (in combination) Janice Duncan

EMERGENCY CARE MANUAL

D0732262

A SYSTEMS APPROACH

Second Edition

by

Burton A. Waisbren, M.D., F.A.C.P.

Associate Director, St. Mary's Hospital Burn Center

Director, Burn Research and Clinical Paradigm Laboratory, St. Mary's Hospital

Member of Intensive Care Comittee, St. Mary's Hospital

Associate Clinical Professor of Medicine, Medical College of Wisconsin

Founding Member of The Society of Critical Care Medicine

Founding Member of The American Burn Association

Member of the Emergency Care Committee, The American Heart Association

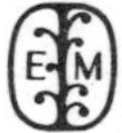
Medical Examination Publishing Co., Inc.
an Excerpta Medica company

Copyright © 1980 by
MEDICAL EXAMINATION
PUBLISHING CO., INC.
an Excerpta Medica company

Library of Congress Card Number
79-91974

ISBN 0-87488-984-7

March, 1980

All rights reserved. No part of this publication may be reproduced in any form or by any means, electronic or mechanical, including photocopy, without permission in writing from the publisher.

Printed in the United States of America

ABOUT THE AUTHOR

Dr. Burton Waisbren's interest in critical care medicine started when, as a boy scout, he was a member of a midwest champion first aid team in 1937. He is now a practicing internist, the Associate Director of St. Mary's Hospital Burn Center in Milwaukee, a member of the American College of Physicians, Clinical Associate Professor of Medicine at the Medical College of Wisconsin, and a founding member of the Infectious Disease Society of America, the American Burn Association, and the Society for Critical Care Medicine. His text on Systems Method for Critical Care Units is widely used throughout the country. He is married and two of his six children have already become physicians.

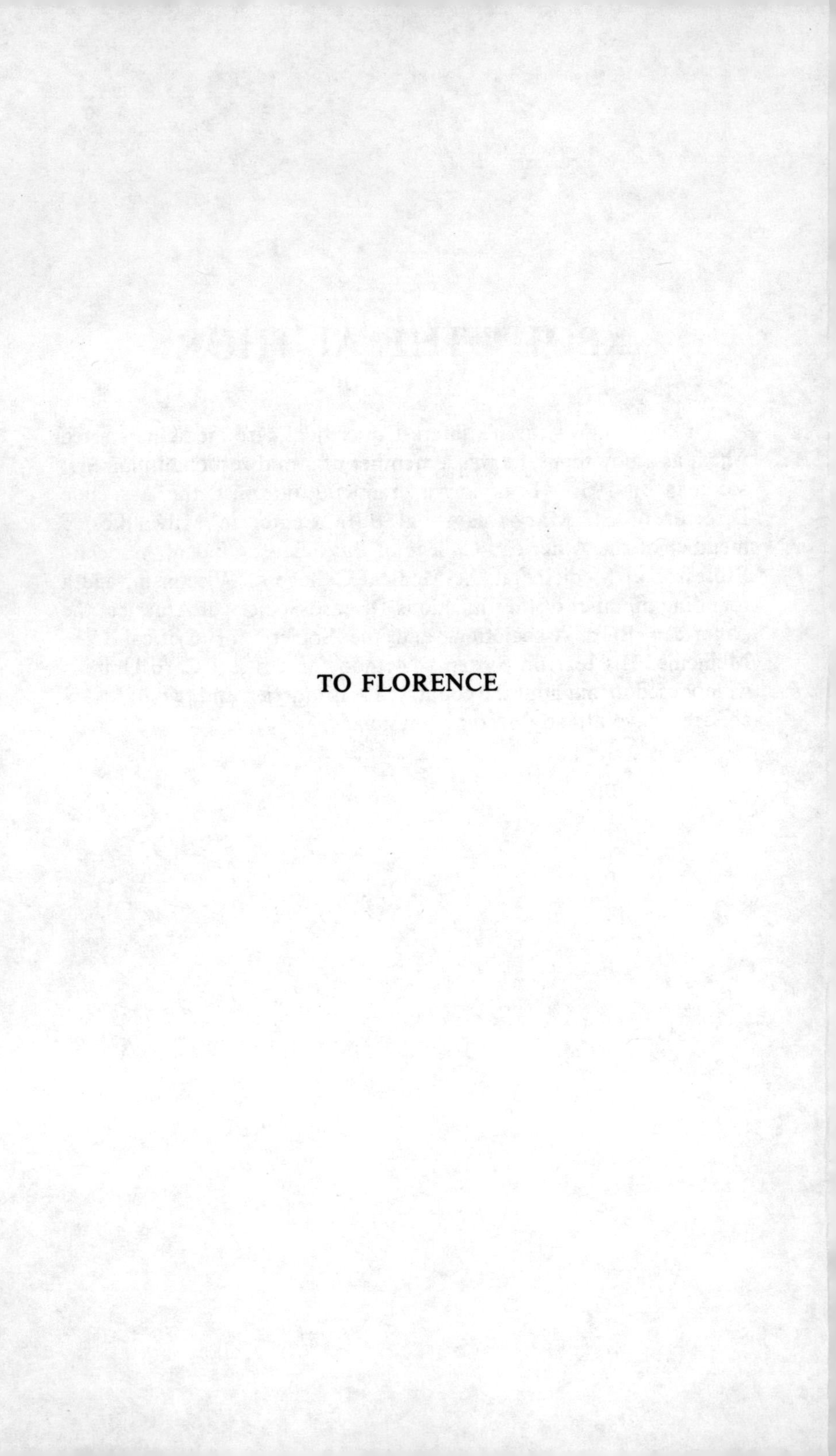

TO FLORENCE

DISCLAIMER

This manual is for TEACHING and INFORMATIONAL use ONLY. ITS FORMAT IS NOT TO BE CONSTRUED AS DIRECTIONS OR AUTHORIZATION FOR ANYONE TO DO ANYTHING IN AN EMERGENCY SITUATION. All opinions expressed are those of the author.

Contents

THE "ANY PORT IN A STORM" PHILOSOPHY

Of course everything in this manual could be done better in a hospital critical care unit by a qualified physician.

The point is that when a person has a **heart attack** or is in a serious **automobile accident**, or when his **heart has stopped**—he rarely is **in** a hospital. As he lies there he will be grateful for "any port in a storm."

The philosophy of this manual is that by **teaching as many people as possible as much as is practicable** the likelihood of the "port" being of genuine help will increase.

This manual I hope will be used to teach nurses, respiratory therapists, physiotherapists, occupational therapists, EKG technicians, paramedics of all degrees, high school students, night school students, and all who want to be able to help in an emergency. I have tried to make it simple enough for all of the above to understand and sophisticated enough to be of true help for the person in distress.

HOW THIS MANUAL MAY BE USED

1. Physicians interested in their patients getting better emergency care may gather together interested people (including ambulance drivers, policepersons, firepersons, teachers, security guards) and use this manual as a text to teach them emergency care. They may then authorize them to do as much as they feel is indicated and legal.
2. Any of the groups mentioned above who see the overt need for the knowledge imparted in this manual and who see the time coming when not only will they be allowed to do more but when they will be expected to be able to act more definitely will contact physicians in their community or people in their community colleges and ask that they be taught the material in this manual.
3. A community unit may feel it wants the protection of better trained emergency personnel and with this manual in hand might be able to bring their local medical society and their community college or high school and their emergency personnel together.

Time after time in this manual we defer to the opinions and preferences of those whom we call the **directing physicians**. Therefore without local interested physicians to help, this manual cannot reach its potential for helping sick or injured people get the best available immediate help.

Ample room is provided throughout for local opinions. On the "Directing Physician" pages which are opposite each system, specific questions often are asked in regard to how the physicians who are teaching the course would prefer to have their patients handled in a particular situation.

INTRODUCTION

This manual came about from a chance encounter in the hospital lobby with an ambulance owner who asked me if I would teach a group of ambulance drivers lifesaving. There seemed to be a genuine desire by the young people concerned for more knowledge regarding what they should do for the patients they were called upon to transport, so I agreed to develop a course with the express purpose of helping emergency personnel to save lives and bring their patients to the hospital in better condition. The drivers concerned all had had the local emergency medical technician courses and were not completely satisfied with them.

Reflection revealed that the stumbling block to the actual saving of lives by emergency personnel was their not being encouraged to convert potentially fatal heart arrhythmias by electrical shock, their not being encouraged to start intravenous fluids, and their not being directed to use emergency drugs. Correcting these deficiencies was made the basic goal of this course. Milwaukee is a typical midwestern community and the announcement of our curriculum caused some adverse reaction from the "establishment." Most threatened seemed those who planned to have a unified emergency care system pointed in the direction of the county hospital. So to avoid confrontations and to get on with the business of saving lives we adopted the ploy of *simulated lifesaving*, that is, all training and systems developed in the initial course and in this book are simulated and can be practiced on make-believe patients. The theory is that when enough personnel have been trained to convert ventricular arrhythmias, to start lifesaving intravenous fluids, and to administer lifesaving drugs, a way will be found to allow them to use their knowledge.

The manual should be used by emergency personnel in conjunction with the physicians who are in actual charge of the patients they are attending. The blank pages after many of the Systems pages are for the modification in the Systems that these physicians may wish to make. We do not dream—nor think that it would be good—for all physicians to treat the situations as we do. However, with a well delineated System to work with most physicians will find it easy to make the modifications they desire.

The manual has been built up in twenty sessions of a course that was given at a community hospital. It starts with a "jump kit." This is based on the premise that even if physicians in your area do not want to authorize you to do anything at the start, the availability of the "jump kit" at the scene of an emergency will allow them to save lives when they arrive to find adequate equipment and medications at hand. After a few such experiences, hopefully they will suggest you go into action even before they are at the scene.

The second section, on Systems, is set up for teaching sessions and discussions. Modifying each System to fit into the opinions of your Directing Physician should help you understand the problems involved.

The third section consists of playlets and contests which we have found to be helpful devices to fix knowledge through competition and variety of approach.

The short EKG course and flash cards are from a course I gave medical students for many years and by practicing with the flash cards you can soon know most of what you need to know about EKG reading for you to react correctly in most situations.

This manual would not have been possible without the diligent and innovative help of my loyal secretary, Mrs. Enid Reichert. I was helped in the teaching of the pilot course by Dr. Burton Friedman, Cardiologist; Dr. Carl Levinson, Obstetrics and Gynecology; Dr. David Altman, Trauma Surgeon; Dr. Walter Shapiro, Internist; and Dr. Lawrence Howards, Anesthesiologist. Many of their ideas are incorporated into the body of the manual and their help is gratefully acknowledged.

The cooperation, enthusiasm, and diligence of the following men, who constituted the pilot project course, also are gratefully acknowledged. They are:

James Baker, Jr., Curtis-Universal Ambulance Co.
Charles Conway, New Berlin Fire Chief
James Baker, Sr., Curtis-Universal Ambulance Co.
James Barnes, New Berlin Fire Department
Joseph Brannan, Wauwatosa Fire Department
Ronald Burghaus, New Berlin Fire Department
Clifford Doerr, New Berlin Fire Department
Robert Heck, New Berlin Fire Department
Richard Forster, New Berlin Fire Department
Gabe King, Curtis-Universal Ambulance Co.
Richard Michalek, New Berlin Fire Department
Richard Plant, West Milwaukee Police Department
Andy Schkeryantz, New Berlin Fire Department
Joseph Wehner, New Berlin Fire Department
Rick Zehetner, Curtis-Universal Ambulance Co.

PREFACE TO SECOND EDITION

The popular acceptance of this manual has been very gratifying. The manual has been completely rewritten to provide the latest information available. It is a pleasure to acknowledge the valuable help and counsel of Dr. Burton A. Waisbren, Jr., Cardiologist, in the revision of this manual. Certainly, since the first edition, a viable alternative to the often excessively long and detailed traditional EMT certification courses has become even more needed. A group learning the material in this manual should be more able to compete with anyone in the field and I hope they will issue challenges where in simulated lifesaving contests they can test their knowledge against their competitors. The public and perhaps the taxpayers will be the real winners.

The diligence and help of my associate, Ms. Diane Schutz, in getting together this new edition is gratefully acknowledged.

JUMP KIT
The Minimum Equipment for an Adequate Emergency Vehicle

CONTENTS AND EXPLANATION

JUMP KIT*

Suction machine—battery operated (Laerdal Corp.)
Pharyngeal airway
Endotracheal tube and laryngoscope
McGill forceps
Emergency tracheostomy needle
Esophageal airway intubation tube

Intravenous set with stand and instructions for use
Disposable sterile stylets for finger pricks
Blood sugar finger prick stops
#14 gage needle with valve for tension pneumothorax
Defibrillator with heart monitor—visual and readout (Get one with capacity of at least 600 milliseconds and preferably 800-1000 for obese patients.)
EKG machine with telephone hookup adaptor, needle, cardiac administration, general administration, needle holder and suture kit
Scalpel—sterile, disposable
Scissors—surgical
Syringes—five 3cc with needles; two 12 cc without needle, two 35 cc without needle

Tape

Tissue Forceps

*There are many good jump kits on the market. For comparison, look at the one put out by Banyan International Corporation, P.O. Box 1779, Abilene, Texas 79604. This has most of the things we have suggested in a compact case.

THE STETHOSCOPE

A stethoscope does away with the necessity of trying to feel the pulse, which is often difficult in the seriously ill or injured. If you do not hear the heartbeat through the stethoscope when it is placed over the left nipple or under the breast (which should be lifted up in obese women), the heart has stopped and you had better go into action.

TO USE THE STETHOSCOPE

Place the diaphragm just below and outside of the nipple in a male. In a female, if the breasts are large lift the left breast and listen just below it. Practice this on your wife so you will not be flustered.

The ear pieces of the stethoscope should be pointed *forward* and placed in your ears—gently. If practice on a number of people has made you familiar with heart sounds, and if you place the stethoscope correctly on the patient's chest and hear nothing—the heart has probably *stopped* and you should start immediate *external cardiac massage* (page 120), and have a member of the team prepare to give a jolt with the defibrillator.

This should be your first action on an unconscious patient because if the heart has *stopped* (and the stethoscope is the best way to find this out) *external cardiac massage* given immediately is the vital thing for you to do (simultaneously checking the airway).

Do not waste time fumbling for a pulse. At the level of this manual, *listen to the heart with a stethoscope to answer only one question*—**is the heart beating or not?**

Do not get a cheap plastic stethoscope, they are hard to hear through.

BLOOD PRESSURE CUFF (SPHYGMOMANOMETER)

The principle of the blood pressure cuff (its fancy name is sphygmomanometer) is simple. The pressure pumped up in the cuff is measured by a spring or mercury manometer and when you fail to hear the heart beat in the antecubital space (the crook of the elbow) when the arm is outstretched, the cuff has achieved a pressure sufficient to equalize the pressure generated by the heart in the artery that runs down the arm.

To "take" the blood pressure you pump up the pressure to 180 and then let the air out of the cuff gradually while listening for heart beats through your stethoscope, whose diaphragm you place at the crook of the elbow. When you hear the first *thumps*, look at the pressure gage and the pressure recorded there is the **systolic blood pressure**. When the sound disappears, note the pressure again. That is the **diastolic pressure**.

If the systolic pressure is over 250, turn to page 40 for the hypertensive crisis system. If, which will be more common, the pressure is under 100—that is, if you do not hear anything at the crook of the elbow until the gage reads less than 100, the patient is probably in shock (if he is ill or had an accident; some normal people have pressures in this range) and turn to page 90 for what your reaction should be.

All interested readers of this manual should buy a blood pressure apparatus (sphygmomanometer) and a stethoscope. Practice with them both with your family so that your spouse and children get used to listening to hearts and taking blood pressures. As you practice taking blood pressures, you might find that some are over 160. If you do, you would be doing that person a favor by telling him or her to see his or her physician for a blood pressure check.

BAG MASK WITH O_2 HOOKUP

Of equal priority to getting the heart to beat is seeing to it that the patient is getting air into the lungs. A **bag mask** (Laerdal Ambo-bag) is the most efficient way to do this and is to be preferred over mouth-to-mouth respiration, which a member of the team should do while you are getting the bag set up and turning on the oxygen tank that it comes with.

Invite an anesthesiologist to teach you how to use the "Ambo-bag" which is his stock and trade. He will demonstrate and amplify the following instructions.

Grab the jaws and lift the neck back. Open the mouth and scoop the back of the throat with your index finger (so you get bitten once in a while) and then place the mask over the nose and mouth and hold it in place with your hand.

With the free hand press the **bag** rhythmically at 14 beats per minute. Coordinate your **bag** breathing with the man doing **external cardiac massage** at a ratio of five chest pressures to one squeeze of the bag.

If you have O_2, hook up 100% to the bag and use that. If you do not, room air is satisfactory.

Practice teaching other people **bag breathing** (it won't hurt your family to know this also) because a bystander will often have to be pressed into service as the "**bag** man."

In the absence of a **bag mask**, mouth-to-mouth resuscitation should be used (see page 121 for instructions on how to do mouth-to-mouth breathing). However, the **bag** attached to an oxygen tank is far superior to mouth-to-mouth breathing.

THE AIRWAY KIT

The **Airway Kit** consists of:
Suction Machine (battery operated) (Laerdal Corp.); **Pharyngeal Airway; Endotracheal Tube; Esophageal Airway Apparatus; Emergency Tracheostomy Needle** (available from Argon Medical Corp., 2612 National Circle Drive, Garland, Texas 75041)

HOW TO USE THE AIRWAY KIT

Finger: Start with the *finger* and scoop out anything you can at the base of the tongue (if this makes the patient vomit be sure to turn his head to one side).
Arms: If the back of the throat is clear to the finger and the airway is still not clear, try the "Heimlich Maneuver" on pages 16–17.

SUCTION MACHINE

Use this with a relatively large rubber tube and check for patency with a cup of water frequently (practice with this machine until you can empty a can of vegetable soup easily).

PHARYNGEAL AIRWAY

The **Pharyngeal Airway** is put in when the back of the throat (the pharynx) is clear. Open the mouth and slip in the airway the easiest way it will go in. This is usually sideways until it is in over the tongue. Then straighten it out. Remove any false teeth (i.e. *removable* false teeth) and save them. Be sure to get a receipt for them when you arrive at the hospital.

McGILL FORCEPS

This is a forceps especially designed to remove foreign bodies such as steak from the throat that you cannot get with your finger or that will be dislodged with the Heimlich Maneuver (pages 16–17). Have a physician who specializes in nose and throat teach you how to use this forceps. That will be the doctor who took out your children's tonsils.

THE LARYNGOSCOPE AND ENDOTRACHEAL TUBE

The **Laryngoscope** and **Endotracheal Tube** are the most complicated and dangerous pieces of equipment in your jump kit and you may decide just to keep it there for a physician to use. However, with practice on a mannequin that has a larynx and after an hour of instruction by an anesthesiologist I feel you can master enough technique for an emergency. Here you can decide between this and your emergency tracheostomy needle.

To insert the **Endotracheal Tube** (Figure 1), slide the **Laryngoscope** in from left to right with the light on, go just beyond the epiglottis (which you will recognize from your mannequin practice) and the vocal cords will be visible. Put the **Endotracheal Tube** into the correct slot in the **Laryngoscope** which will guide it into the trachea (the trachea is the large tube that runs from the back of the pharynx into the bronchial tubes, which are the large air passages of the lungs). Then instill some water into the small balloon that collars the **Endotracheal Tube** and gives it an airtight fit. Then hook up the oxygen and breathe the patient with your Ambo-bag. Suction the tube if it gets noisy. Once the tube is in, keep reassuring the patient, who will think you are choking him to death. At this point some morphine will be particularly helpful and safe, since you can breathe for the patient if it depresses his respirations. You should practice this procedure under supervision weekly on your mannequin designed for this. **This mannequin is a "must" for any group serious about saving lives at the scene of an accident or emergency.**

EMERGENCY TRACHEOSTOMY NEEDLE

This needle is stuck into the midline just below the "Adam's apple" and has a curve downward. A syringe fits onto it and will aspirate the tracheal well. Then the needle will accept an O_2 catheter and allow for controlled breathing using the Ambo-bag. Certainly this is an excellent alternative to inserting an endotracheal tube and your jump kit must leave both options open (Figure 2).

ESOPHAGEAL AIRWAY

This device works by having you place a tube in the stomach, then having you blow a balloon that shuts off the stomach from the esophagus so that if you blow oxygen into the pharynx via either the nose or mouth the oxygen will end up in the lungs rather than the stomach. This is rather inefficient and a third option after the emergency tracheostomy needle and the endotracheal tube.

CORRECT

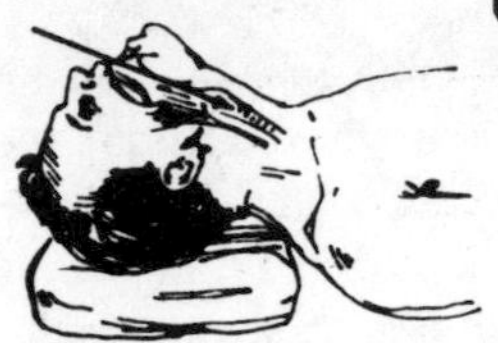

Neck should be flexed, head extended and supported on pillow to bring mouth, larnyx and trachea in line

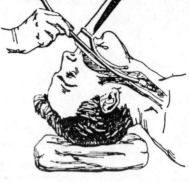

Endotracheal tube introduced with laryngoscope 3 or 4 cm past glottis

INCORRECT

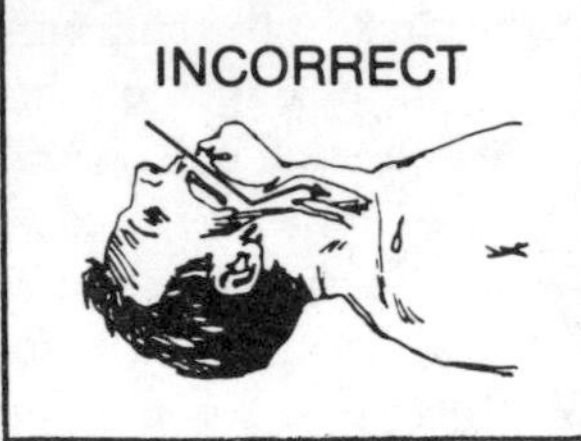

VOCAL CORDS OPEN

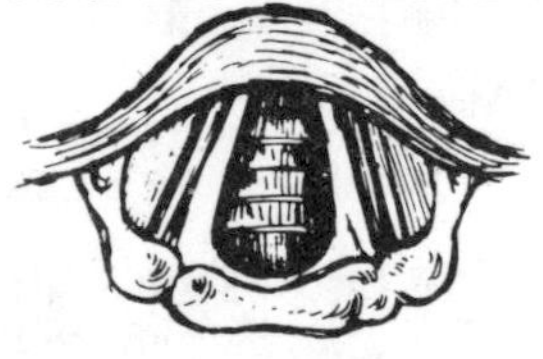

VOCAL CORDS CLOSED

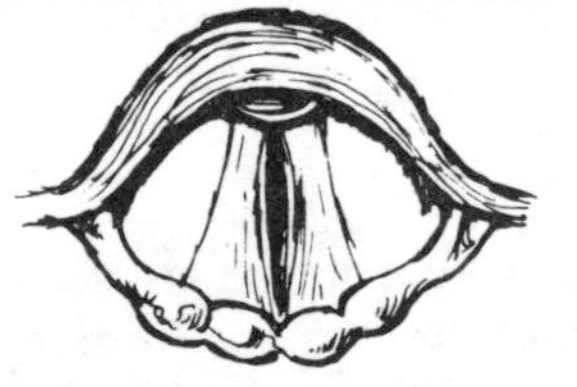

1. Extend neck or elevate head.
2. Insert laryngoscope and elevate tongue.
3. Look for esophagus posterior and vocal cords and epiglottis anterior.
4. Place endotracheal tube through (between) vocal cords.

   Caution: Intubation should not be attempted when glottis is closed because of trauma to vocal cords.
5. Check by blowing through endotracheal tube and watch for chest movements.
6. Listen for breath sounds — avoid placing tube in esophagus.
7. Inflate balloon (cuff) of endotracheal tube to obtain good seal.

Figure 1. Insertion of endotracheal tube.

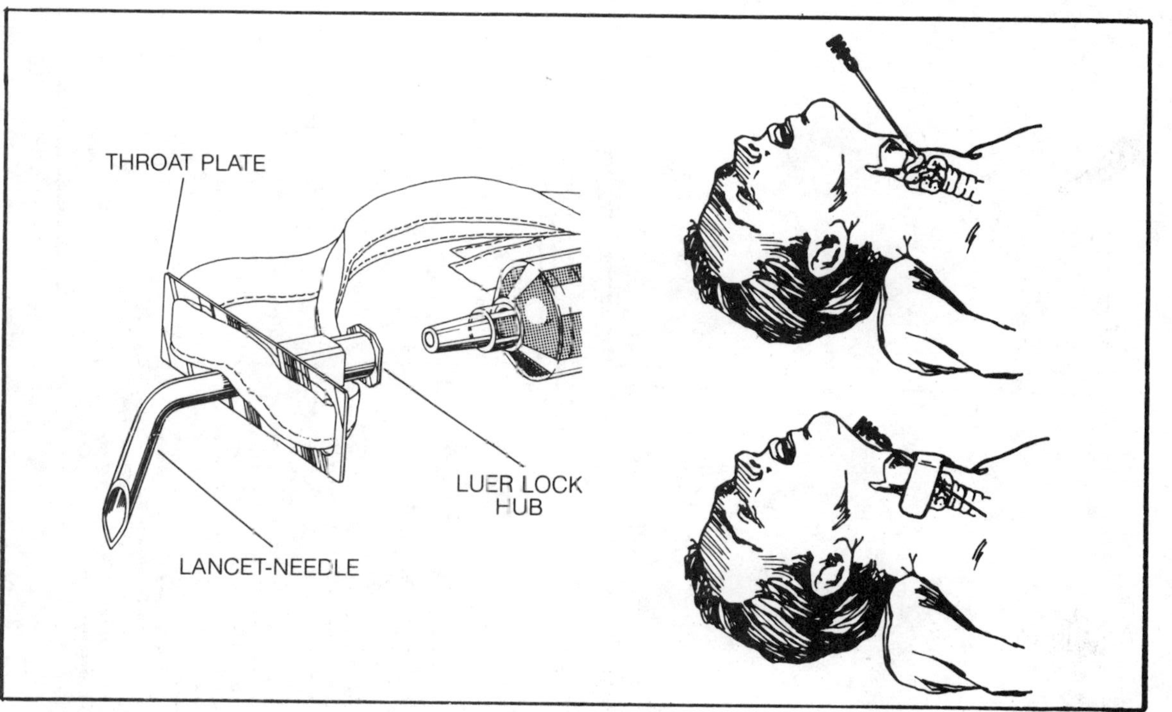

Figure 2. Emergency tracheostomy needle.

THE HEIMLICH MANEUVER

The basic technique

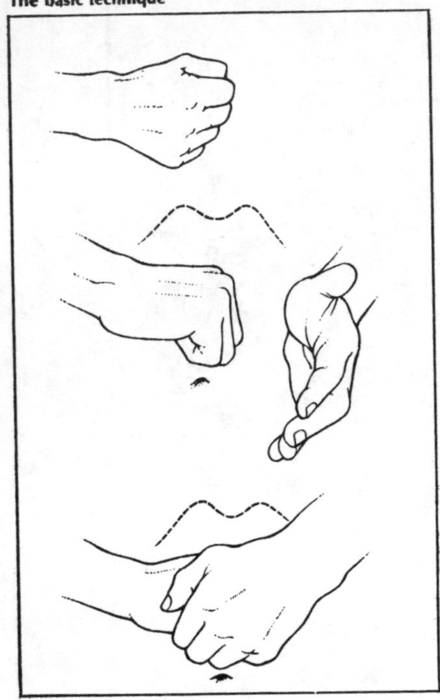

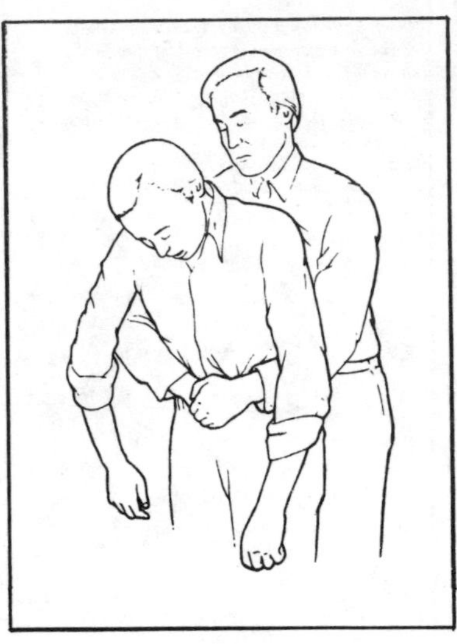

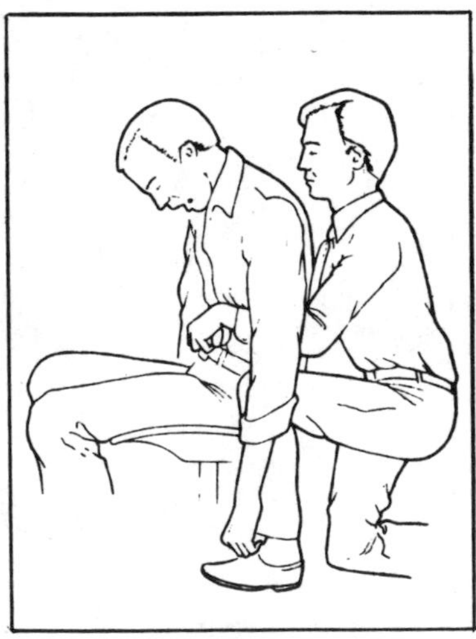

The maneuver devised by Dr. Henry J. Heimlich, professor of advanced clinical sciences at Xavier University in Cincinnati, uses air in the lungs to force an obstruction out of the airway. To move the air you have to apply sudden pressure below the rib cage, which forces the diaphragm up and compresses the lungs. The basic technique (above) begins with a fist. Note the knob formed by the thumb and index finger—that's what helps push the diaphragm upward. Place your fist thumbside against the abdomen, slightly above the navel and below the rib cage. Then grasp your fist with your free hand and press into the abdomen with a quick upward thrust. Do this while standing or kneeling behind a standing or sitting victim with your arms wrapped around his waist (right). Repeat this procedure several times if necessary.

Reprinted with permission from: *Emergency Medicine.* Copyright© by Merk & Co., Inc.

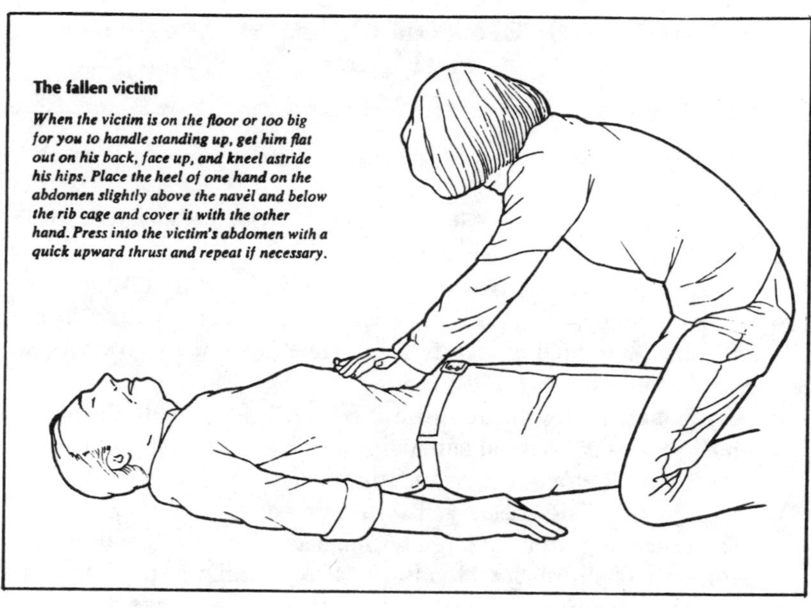
The fallen victim
When the victim is on the floor or too big for you to handle standing up, get him flat out on his back, face up, and kneel astride his hips. Place the heel of one hand on the abdomen slightly above the navel and below the rib cage and cover it with the other hand. Press into the victim's abdomen with a quick upward thrust and repeat if necessary.

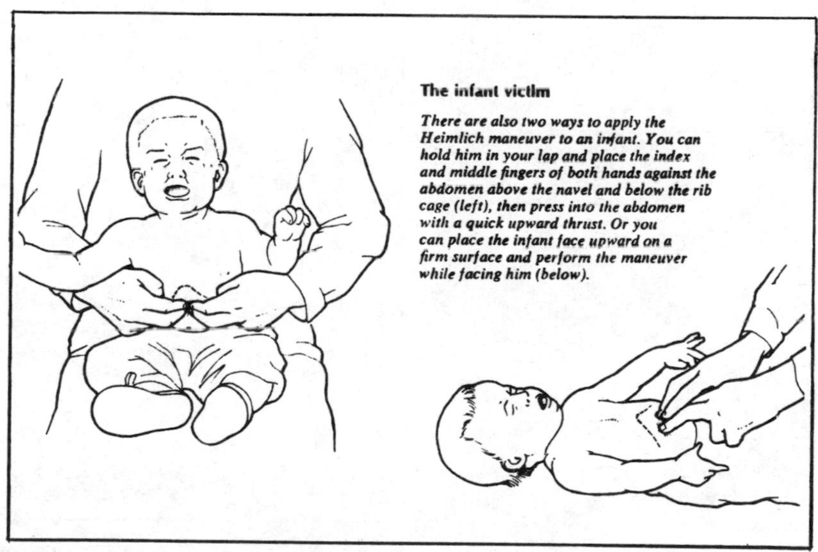
The infant victim
There are also two ways to apply the Heimlich maneuver to an infant. You can hold him in your lap and place the index and middle fingers of both hands against the abdomen above the navel and below the rib cage (left), then press into the abdomen with a quick upward thrust. Or you can place the infant face upward on a firm surface and perform the maneuver while facing him (below).

Reprinted with permission from: *Emergency Medicine*. Copyright© by Merk & Co., Inc.

FOUR TOURNIQUETS FOR BLEEDING AND HEART FAILURE

Tourniquets are, of course, to stop **arterial bleeding** in the extremities.

Mine Safety Appliance Kit tourniquets or triangle bandages with a stick for tightening are suggested.

Remember, however, that *pressure* over the area is still the best way to stop bleeding—arterial or venous. Take a sterile pad or clean handkerchief and hold as tightly as possible over the involved area. This will stop most arterial bleeding.

If you **do use a tourniquet—use it correctly—tighten to the point at which you see the arterial pumping stop.** Get an opinion from your own Directing Physician regarding **tourniquets**. I think you will find most surgeons would **prefer you to use pressure.**

The other important use for **tourniquets** is to trap blood in the extremities to help reduce blood return to a failing heart. For this reason also, they must be part of the jump kit (see page 88).

THE FIRST AID KIT

The standard Mine Safety Appliance Kit used by most fire departments is one of many satisfactory first aid kits and is readily available. It has bandages, triangular bandages, and dressings that will cover most situations. Add to it items it does not have that are mentioned on page 8. In addition, add a prepackaged obstetrical kit which you can get from the Central Supply department at your hospital.

Splints should be chosen by the orthopedic physicians in your community.

We have been impressed with the spine board diagrammed in Figure 3. If your group is apt to be involved in spine injuries, I would suggest you have one made or make it yourself. It was designed by "Pinkey" Newell of Purdue University and was first published in the excellent magazine, *Emergency Medicine*.

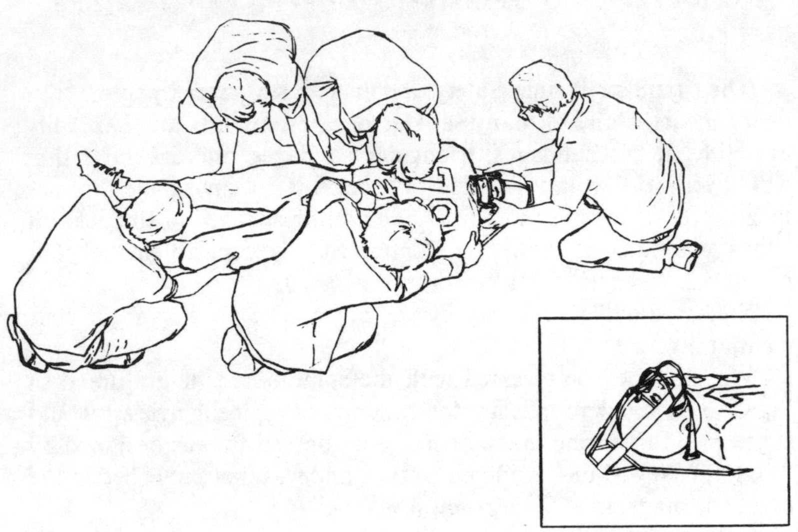

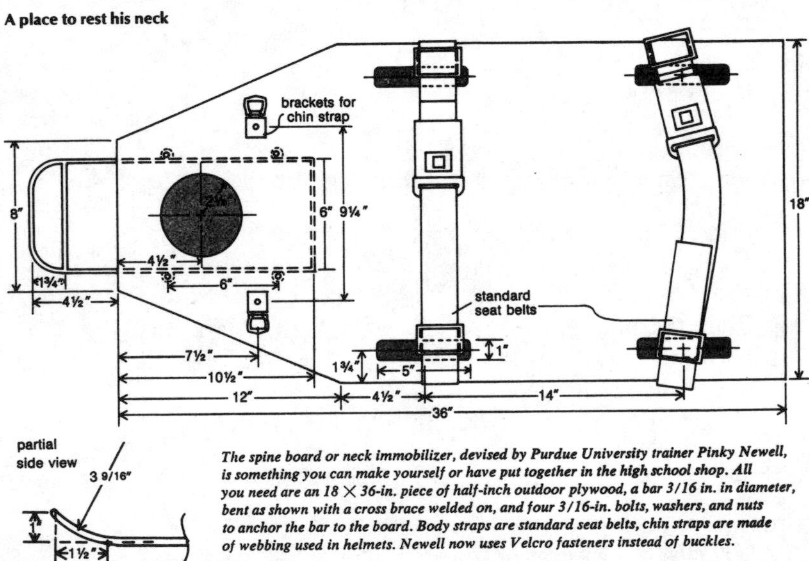

The spine board or neck immobilizer, devised by Purdue University trainer Pinky Newell, is something you can make yourself or have put together in the high school shop. All you need are an 18 × 36-in. piece of half-inch outdoor plywood, a bar 3/16 in. in diameter, bent as shown with a cross brace welded on, and four 3/16-in. bolts, washers, and nuts to anchor the bar to the board. Body straps are standard seat belts, chin straps are made of webbing used in helmets. Newell now uses Velcro fasteners instead of buckles.

Figure 3. The spine board. Reprinted with permission from: *Emergency Medicine*. Copyright© by Merk & Co., Inc.

INTRAVENOUS STAND AND INTRAVENOUS SET

FLUID FOR INTRAVENOUS ADMINISTRATION

There are many of these available and we suggest you use the standard brand of Ringer's Lactate* that is used in your local hospital's emergency room. This solution has salt (NaCl) and potassium and is the standard I.V. fluid for almost all situations you might encounter. Bleeding, diabetic coma, severe burn, shock, and drug ingestion all are treated best with intravenous Ringer's Lactate. How rapidly the fluid should be run in is indicated in the specific Systems sections of this manual. This is determined by counting the number of drops per minute as seen in the "dropping chamber" of the I.V. set.

Being willing to start and administer intravenous fluids is the *sine qua non* of true emergency care and trying to help without this capability (and the willingness to administer drugs and electric shock) makes emergency care a charade.

TECHNIQUE FOR STARTING AN I.V.

Have initial instruction by a physician and then arrange for more help at the emergency rooms to which you will be transporting your patient. An excellent I.V. mannequin arm is available for constant practice.

1. Have the patient lying down with collar open.
2. Have the patient's arm exposed well above the elbow.
3. Place the adaptor set and tubing in the indicated place in the stopper of the I.V. bottle (not in the air vent) and let the solution run out of the needle, being sure all the air is out of the tubing. (People get hysterical about leaving a little air in the tube, but the fact

*Content of one liter Ringer's Lactate (Hartman's osolution) is:
130 mEq of sodium
4 mEq of potassium
3 mEq of calcium
109 mEq of chloride
28 mEq of lactate

is that a few bubbles of air are not going to hurt anything.) When you have fluid running out of the needle, close the clamp on the tubing that regulates fluid rate and put the cap over your needle.

4. Wipe off the entire inner aspect of the elbow with an alcohol sponge.
5. Place a tourniquet above the elbow, halfway up the arm, and fairly tight. This should cause veins to bulge at the crook of the patient's elbow. The veins look like rubber tubes underneath the skin.
6. Taking care not to touch the skin, place the needle, bevel up, into the vein. If the needle is in the vein you will see blood run back into the tubing. As soon as you do, release the tourniquet around the patient's arm and the clamp that regulates flow of the I.V. The fluid will then flow steadily into the viewing chamber of the I.V. set. Regulate the flow into this chamber by tightening the clamp above it to deliver the required drops per minute.

I believe it is safe and worthwhile for the members of an emergency care course to start I.V.s on each other under the direction of a physician. Once you have done some on yourselves, you may be allowed to help do this in an emergency ward.

TABLE TO CONVERT DROPS/MIN TO CC OR ML/HOUR

Total Fluid Per Hour	Drops Per Minute Needed
100 cc/hour	16 drops/min
250 cc/hour	40 drops/min
500 cc/hour	80 drops/min
1000 cc/hour	160 drops/min

BLOOD SUGAR FINGER PRICK STICKS*

These small sticks should allow you to diagnose and start treatment of **diabetic coma** and **insulin reaction** (pages 84 and 116).

The test should be done on any unconscious patient (**not** at the cost, however, of a delay in transit).

To do the test, milk the finger and trap the blood at the tip. Wipe the finger with an alcohol sponge. Prick the finger with a disposable stylet or sterile needle. Place a drop of blood on the stick, let it stay for 60 seconds, wash it off with the wash bottle provided with the set and match the color standard to determine the concentration of sugar in the drop of blood tested.

If the **blood sugar** is **below 50, you probably are dealing with insulin overdosage** and I.V. 50% glucose is indicated immediately (page 116).

If the **blood sugar** is **over 250**—you may be dealing with **diabetic coma**. If you wish to be more precise, buy the small portable machine that reads these sticks accurately up to blood sugars of 1000. If you have this machine you will know blood sugars over 500 and be able to give insulin along with fluid (page 44).

It is rarely necessary for you to determine blood sugars on patients who are conscious.

Practice determining blood sugar by this method on each other and/or your family. You might even find a case of early diabetes, i.e. blood sugar over 150.

*The blood sugar prick sticks with excellent instructions are available from Ames Chemical Company, Ames, Iowa.

#14 GAGE NEEDLE WITH VALVE FOR TENSION PNEUMOTHORAX

Tension pneumothorax will be discussed under System for chest injury (page 100), so suffice it to say that when a penetrating injury to the chest wall sucks in air which then cannot get out, this can be relieved by this valved #14 needle. The #14 gage needle is inserted inward and downward at the middle of the scapula (collar bone); you push in until you hear the air escape through the valve. The device will then act as a safety valve so that air being sucked into the lung cannot build up pressure that will compromise breathing.

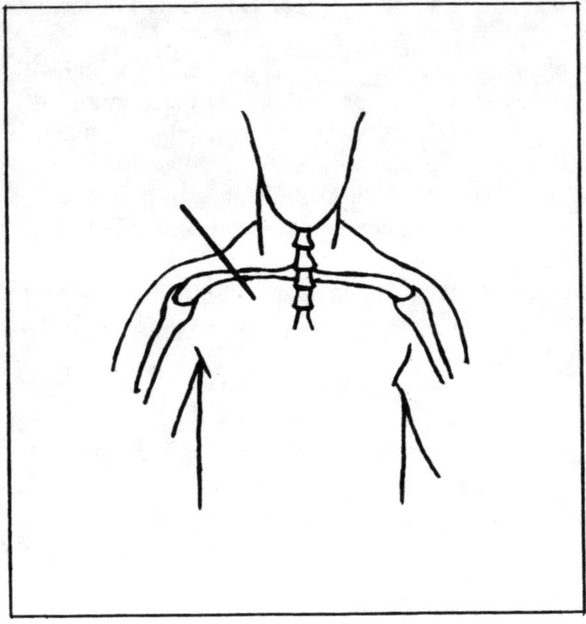

Figure 4.

URINARY CATHETER SET

These are all made up and can be obtained from the Central Supply department of your local hospital. There is nothing more disconcerting or painful than the time someone gets acute urinary retention after drinking too much beer at a picnic or when for the first time his prostate gland reaches the time of obstruction. Having a catheter set up in the emergency vehicle will often prevent a hospital visit in that a physician or nurse can "catch" the patient and then perhaps take care of the situation in the morning.

The alternative procedure is to use a 30 cc syringe and the cardiac injection needle and draw out urine by inserting the needle directly in the midline at the pubis—which is the front bone of the pelvis—start feeling at the umbilicus (belly button) and go directly down until you feel the bone and insert the needle there, after wiping off the area with an alcohol sponge. There are no vital organs there and urine will spill out from the distended bladder. Your instructor can show you how to do this in ten minutes.

NOTES

Drugs to Stock and Use for Emergency Care

At a minimum these should be available for use by a physician who might arrive at the scene of an accident.

Ideally, the physicians who direct the course as outlined in this book will authorize those of you who demonstrate the proper knowledge, maturity, and judgment to give the drugs as outlined in the following pages. How this idea will work out in practice will have to be decided locally between emergency personnel and physicians who direct them. My opinion in this regard is expressed in the "port in a storm" remarks.

DRUGS TO BE STOCKED

Keep the package inserts in each package and review them before giving the drug.

No. to Stock	Drug	Use	Page
	Adrenalin	Acute asthma	32
4	1 cc amps, 1:1000	Acute allergic reaction	
6	1:10,000 dilution in prefilled syringe	Cardiac arrest	
	Aminophyllin	Acute asthma	33
3	10 cc amps (250 mg), 3–3/4 gr also in predrawn syringes		
	Amytal	Uncontrolled seizures	34
3	10 cc amps, 3–3/4 gr	Epilepsy	
	Atropine	Slow heart after attack	35
3	1 mg/1 cc amps	Severe chest pains	
	Compazine	Intractable vomiting	36
3	2 cc amps, 10 mg		
	*Demerol**	Severe pain of heart attack or ruptured ulcer	37
*	1 cc amps, 75 mg		
	Dextrose 5%	Insulin reaction	38
4	50 cc bottle or prefilled syringe		
	Diazoxide (Hyperstat)	Blood pressure over 250	40
3	20 ml amps, 300 mg		
	Digoxin (Lanoxin)	Superventricular tachycardia	41
4	2 cc amps, 0.5 mg		
	Dopamine	Cardiogenic shock	42
1	5 cc amps, 200 mg		
	Ergotrate	Uterine hemorrhage	43
4	1/300 gr amps		
4	*Glucagon*	Insulin reaction	39
	1 mg/cc vials		

*Do not stock this. Explain in large letters that drugs you keep on an emergency vehicle do not include narcotics.

DRUGS TO BE STOCKED (Continued)

No. to Stock	Drug	Use	Page
	Insulin, regular	Diabetic coma	44
2	100 units per cc—**refrigerated**		
	Lasix	Heart failure	45
2	40 mg vials		
	Narcan	Drug overdose,	46
4	2 cc amps	narcotic	
	Nitroglycerine	Heart pain	47
1	100 tablet bottles		
	Propranolol (Inderal)	Heart arrhythmia	48
5	1 mg/1 ml amps	Chest pain	
	Reactose Gel (Glutose)	Insulin reaction	49
2	2 oz. bottles	Try in coma	
	Ringer's Lactate	Cardiogenic shock	50
2	500 cc bottles	Blood loss	
		Diabetic coma	
	Sodabicarb ($NaHCO_3$)	After cardiac arrest	51
9	50 cc vials	Diabetic coma	
	Also in prefilled syringes		
	Solu-Cortef	Impending death	52
2	2 cc Mix-O-Vials, 500 mg	Status asthmaticus	
	Valium	Extreme anxiety	53
5	10 mg	D.T.s	
	Also in prefilled syringes		
	Xylocaine 2%	Cardiac arrhythmias	54
2	5 cc amps, 20 mg/cc		
6	75 mg prefilled syringes		

NOTES

About the Drugs

The following section is not meant to be a pharmacology text, but rather to share with you the pertinent information about the drugs you will have available that I feel will be the most helpful to you to review just before you use the medication. Remember, authorization to use these drugs cannot come from this manual. This is a matter between you and a Directing Physician.

ADRENALIN

HOW SUPPLIED

1:1000, 1 cc ampules; 1:10,000 dilution in prefilled syringe with 3-1/2 inch needle for intracardiac administration

USUAL DOSE

1 cc for acute asthma or allergic reaction; 2 cc for cardiac arrest

CAPSULE COMMENT

This is a powerful natural stimulant. One cc given subcutaneously will often miraculously help a patient with a severe asthmatic attack. It may start a stopped heart if used as directed on page 71. Its action is very rapidly over and there is very little danger in giving almost anyone a shot of adrenalin for asthma (page 109) or an acute anaphylactic shock (page 118).

SOME SPECIFICS

Heart Attack: If you come upon a heart attack victim whose heart has stopped, inject 2 cc adrenalin with a long needle into the heart. Go upward and inward and toward the middle from the nipple, aiming for the right ear if the patient is lying on his back. Don't be shy—the patient has nothing to lose. **Do not delay external cardiac massage** while this is being prepared.

If no response, try again. If still no response, keep external massage and then try a **shock** (400 watt sec) for at least six times.

CAUTION: Adrenalin causes heart arrhythmia, so be sure the heart is really *stopped* (stethoscope) before you put it into someone's chest!

Acute Bronchial Asthma: You will rarely see an asthmatic in real trouble with the first attack. If he says he is an asthmatic he probably is, and if he seems in really acute distress and has blue nail beds—give him one cc of adrenalin into the external aspect of his arm.

CAUTION: Elderly people may be having **cardiac** asthma, so only use it in patients over 60 if you are assured he has chronic **bronchial** asthma that has responded to adrenalin in the past.

AMINOPHYLLIN

HOW SUPPLIED

10 cc ampules, 250 mg. (3–3/4 gr)
also available in prefilled syringes

USUAL DOSE

250 mg I.V.

CAPSULE COMMENT

This given intravenously, slowly, will often help asthmatics who no longer respond to adrenalin. Give it slowly over a period of 5 minutes if the patient seems just unable to stop wheezing. Then put another 3-3/4 grains in the 500 cc of lactate that you give slowly during transport.

AMYTAL

HOW SUPPLIED

10 cc ampule, 3–3/4 gr

USUAL DOSE

5 ml I.M.
I.V. injection not to exceed 1 ml/min; maximum single dose 1 gram (adult); 10% solution with sterile water

CAPSULE COMMENT

This is a barbiturate that may be necessary to stop severe convulsions that occur in continuous epileptic seizures (status epilepticus) or sometimes after a severe stroke. Try to put in a pharyngeal airway when you are forced to use it. If the patient is convulsing too actively for you to start an I.V. give it intramuscularly in the hip.

ATROPINE

HOW SUPPLIED

1 mg/1 cc

USUAL DOSE

1 mg

CAPSULE COMMENT

Atropine inhibits the nerve that slows the heart rate after a heart attack. That is to say the vagus nerve acts as a brake on the heart and when it is slowing the heart *too much* after a heart attack the atropine will allow it to speed up enough to pump enough blood to sustain the patient's blood pressure and life.

INDICATION

A slow heart (under a rate of 60) after a heart attack or severe chest pains (page 78). If the first dose does not speed the heart you may repeat it in 5 minutes. Then use it as necessary when the heart rate starts to slow once again or at one-half hour intervals.

COMPAZINE

HOW SUPPLIED

2 cc ampules; 10 mg

USUAL DOSE

10 mg

CAPSULE COMMENT

Ten mg of Compazine into the buttock will stop most persistent vomiting. It may be repeated hourly. Occasionally the patient will see double from Compazine. If this happens just do not give another dose.

DEMEROL

HOW SUPPLIED

1 cc ampules; 25, 50, 75, 100 mg

USUAL DOSE

50–150 mg I.M. or S.Q.

CAPSULE COMMENT

This is a very potent narcotic pain reliever which should be given to coronary patients. It has almost no danger and may be repeated. Intramuscular injections are best. There is a problem with keeping demerol in a kit since addicts will steal it. Perhaps it would be best to discretely hide some (obtained legally by your Directing Physician) in your emergency vehicle. Perhaps it would be better to try to get along without it. This will have to be decided locally.

INDICATIONS

Severe Chest Pain

This both reassures and relieves the victim of a heart attack.

Severe Injury

The pain relief and reassurance of demerol may prevent the victim of a severe accident from going into shock.

How to Give

One 2 cc disposable ampule, 100 mg given into outer aspect of left arm.

Danger

Chronic lung patients should not be given narcotics unless their pain is terribly intense.

DEXTROSE
(50% GLUCOSE)

HOW SUPPLIED

50 cc bottle, I.V. only
also available in prefilled syringe

USUAL DOSE

See below

CAPSULE COMMENT

This is a miraculous drug when given to a patient in a coma due to an overdose of insulin, and if there is any question of the cause of the coma, 50% glucose should be given intravenously.

Be **very sure** you are in the vein when you use it, because it causes difficulty when it leaks under the skin. Therefore, start a lactated Ringer's I.V. at 20 drops per minute and put the glucose in the I.V. tubing.

Most insulin overdose patients will wake up with one vial. If they lapse off again, give them another vial.

The only toxicity of the 50% glucose occurs when it goes outside the vein, so it should be given when there is even a **remote** possibility of insulin overdose. It will not even hurt a patient in **diabetic coma** (page 84).

GLUCAGON

HOW SUPPLIED

1 mg/cc ampules

USUAL DOSE

0.5–1.0 mg.

CAPSULE COMMENT

Glucagon is the body's way of raising blood sugar and works in a balanced system with insulin (which decreases blood sugar) and therefore it's the logical thing to give for an overdose of insulin as outlined on p. 84.

DIAZOXIDE (HYPERSTAT)

HOW SUPPLIED

20 ml ampules; 300 mg.

USUAL DOSE

See below

CAPSULE COMMENT

This important new medication will rapidly bring down very high blood pressure. If the patient's blood pressure is over 250 systolic and the patient is unconscious, give 2 cc (15 mg/cc) intravenously. If the blood pressure then goes below 200 give 2 cc I.V. into the I.V. tubing *every* half hour. If there is no response and the patient is getting worse, try 4 cc I.V. (60 mg.). It has no important toxicity if used as above.

DIGOXIN (LANOXIN)

HOW SUPPLIED

2 cc ampules; 0.5 mg.

USUAL DOSE

1 cc

CAPSULE COMMENT

This heart drug must be considered one of the very dangerous drugs in your kit. However, it is very effective in heart arrhythmias (page 79) and one-half of a cc or one cc given intravenously will often convert a dangerously fast heart and/or help heart failure.

HOW IT WORKS

This is the most controversial drug you will carry in your kit. It is a digitalis preparation that acts rapidly to increase the ability of the heart to beat forcibly. **An overdose will cause the heart to have excess irritability and fatal arrythmia**—so the drug **cannot be used without authorization** and the **full knowledge** that it can easily **kill** the patient. When you **do** give it, a **monitor must be going** and an **I.V. with lidocaine ready.**

DOPAMINE

HOW SUPPLIED

200 mg; 5 cc capsules

USUAL DOSE

200 mg per 500 cc bottle I.V. fluid

CAPSULE COMMENT

This is an adrenalin-like compound. Put the 200 mg vial in the 500 cc of Ringer's Lactate when the systolic blood pressure is below 75 either from cardiogenic shock or from shock from any other cause but bleeding and adjust the I.V. rate (page 22) to keep the systolic blood pressure over 85 and you may often save a life. It should only be used if your Directing Physician* has given this permission in writing.

PRECAUTIONS

Monitor with EKG—if over six ventricular extra beats per minute use Lidocaine with it as outlined on page 54.

Run the I.V. only fast enough to achieve a blood pressure of 100. If at a wide-open rate (100 drops per minute) the blood pressure or heart rate do not respond at all—stop and change to Ringer's Lactate (page 50), running wide-open for an hour without Dopamine.

If the patient does not have obvious chest pains or EKG changes, suspect other causes of shock—most likely a gastrointestinal bleeding. This is treated with the wide-open running Ringer's.

*Some cardiologists do not like Dopamine used in cardiogenic shock.

ERGOTRATE

HOW SUPPLIED

1/300 gr ampule

USUAL DOSE

1 cc

CAPSULE COMMENT

This drug may help you save a life by the fact that it contracts the uterus and stops the bleeding within it, caused by the fact that sometimes the uterus does not contract after childbirth. A woman with a severe uterine hemorrhage after the delivery of a baby should be given 1 cc intravenously.

DOSAGE

Give 1 cc intravenously to a patient with uterine hemorrhage after childbirth or a miscarriage if she is losing blood at a rate that is causing her blood pressure to drop or that is causing her to lose consciousness.

CAUTION

Do not give to a patient in labor. Do not give to a patient who is more than 4 months along in pregnancy.

INSULIN

HOW SUPPLIED

100 units per cc; this must be kept **refrigerated.**

USUAL DOSE

Regular U-100, 10 cc, 50 units I.V. and 50 units S.Q.

CAPSULE COMMENT

Regular insulin may save the life of patient in diabetic coma (page 84).

Rapid administration of Ringer's Lactate is equally important in the coma patient (page 50), so **start the I.V. first in diabetic coma.**

CRITERIA TO BE MET FOR THE GIVING OF INSULIN IN THE AMBULANCE

1. Agreement by the Directing Physician to the following (he can sign this page of the manual to this effect):
2. Patient unconscious or semiconscious.
3. Blood sugar over 300 by finger prick method (page 23).
4. Patient is breathing rapidly and fully.

IF ABOVE CRITERIA MET—THEN GIVE:

50 units of regular insulin I.V. and 50 units subcutaneously (1/2 cc by each route—your Directing Physician may want to halve this dose).

Keep the Ringer's Lactate going at 40 drops per minute—check urine for sugar as often as you can get specimens.

Try to get a history regarding previous diabetes, previous insulin, and anything else unusual that happened to the patient. (Diabetic coma usually has a precipitating cause.) Keep a complete record to give to the admitting ward (page 132).

LASIX

HOW SUPPLIED

40 mg vials
also available in prefilled syringes

USUAL DOSE

1 cc I.V. (40 mg)

CAPSULE COMMENT

The all-purpose diuretic—the emergency situation in which it is most helpful is acute congestive heart failure. Forty mg I.V. will often cause the patient to urinate enough fluid to relieve fluid back-up congestion in his lungs. Lasix has a wide margin of safety (unless the patient is a hypertensive who has been taking medications; do not use Lasix because they are apt to be running too low a potassium level to stand a good diuresis).

NARCAN

HOW SUPPLIED

2 cc

USUAL DOSE

2 cc

CAPSULE COMMENT

This drug acts as a specific antagonist of narcotics. If a coma is due to narcotic overdose, the patient may wake up rapidly after a 2 cc dose of Narcan I.V. (.8 mg). It will not hurt patients in a coma due to other drugs.

USE

Use when you come upon an unconscious patient who has the possibility of an overdose (needle marks on the arm, syringe or pen point nearby) and who is not breathing or is breathing very slowly.

DOSE

Give 2 cc of Narcan (.8 mg.) and the patient may suddenly wake up. If he does and then lapses again, give 2 cc every 1/2 hour until at emergency room.

NITROGLYCERIN TABLETS

HOW SUPPLIED

100 tablet bottle

USUAL DOSE

Sublingually

CAPSULE COMMENT

These are harmless in spite of their awesome name, and should be given under the tongue at 5-minute intervals for patients with cardiac pain (providing their blood pressure stays above 110, systolic).

PROPRANOLOL (INDERAL)

HOW SUPPLIED

1 mg/1 ml ampules

USUAL DOSE

1–3 mg

CAPSULE COMMENT

This is a blocker of stimuli to a specific type of receptors in the sympathetic nervous system. It should be available for emergency care since a physician may direct you to give 1–3 cc (1–3 mg) if other drugs are not controlling a heart arrhythmia or chest pain.

REACTOSE GEL (GLUTOSE)

HOW SUPPLIED

2 oz bottle

USUAL DOSE

One-third of bottle, repeated if necessary

CAPSULE COMMENT

This is a pure, easily absorbable sugar, which will bring a person out of insulin coma if placed in the mouth. It will also prevent coma from insulin should the patient not be able to keep up his food intake after taking his insulin. It is worth squeezing Glutose into the mouth of any unconscious person. He may suddenly wake up.

RINGER'S LACTATE

HOW SUPPLIED

500 cc bottles

USUAL DOSE

See below for specific indications

CAPSULE COMMENT

A universal I.V. fluid that can be used as a vehicle for drugs like Aminophyllin and Dopamine, and perhaps more important will temporarily replace blood volume when a person is suffering or has suffered acute blood loss.

USE

This I.V. fluid has chemicals in it that approximate those in the human plasma. Therefore, it is excellent for restoration of the circulation.

CAUTION: The only danger its use entails is that of overloading the heart with too much fluid. Therefore, **remember**, the **older** the patient or the **worse** his heart, the **less** Ringer's Lactate you use. Practice starting I.V.s with Ringer's Lactate on each other. It is harmless.

PREPARE

Use only an unopened bottle and sealed tubing set that is opened just before use. The I.V. line running with Ringer's Lactate gives you an inlet to inject I.V. medications and also a way of keeping the blood flowing to the organs if the patient is in shock.

SPECIFIC INDICATIONS

Severe burns: 100 cc per hour, at 160 drops/min; **Shock (Blood Loss):** 500 cc per hour, at 80 drops/min; **Acute Bleeding:** At rate to replace blood or raise blood pressure to 100—80 drops/min; **Cardiac Resuscitation:** To use for inlet for medications—Lidocaine, Isuprel, Digoxin—at 20 drops/min; **Diabetic Coma,** 500 cc/hour if under 50 years of age—80 drops/min; **Barbiturate Overdose:** 500 cc/hour—80 drops/min.

If the patient starts to wheeze or complains of difficulty in breathing—*slow the fluid*!

SODABICARB ($NaHCO_3$)

HOW SUPPLIED

50 cc vials
also available in prefilled syringes

USUAL DOSE

1–3 vials

CAPSULE COMMENT

Whenever a person goes into shock or has a severe heart attack with the heart stopping, acid builds up in his system that causes further cellular damage. Thus, anyone in this category should benefit from having this acid neutralized by the immediate injection of one or two ampules of sodabicarbonate. It can do little harm and may do a lot of good.

USE

This prepared vial contains 3-3/4 grams of baking soda. We use it in cases of **shock**, because when the cells do not get enough oxygen they put acid into the blood stream. This in turn causes the heart to become irritable and to go into **ventricular rhythms**—which **may be fatal**. The I.V. baking soda neutralizes this acid and therefore prevents cardiac arrhythmias. It is **always** given intravenously.

DOSE

One vial—moderate shock; 2 vials—worse shock; 3 vials—post-resuscitation.

TOXICITY

This is very safe and any patient in severe shock will benefit from a vial of sodabicarb. Give a vial every hour until patient is in the emergency room if patient has been resuscitated heart-wise but is still not out of the woods.

SOLU-CORTEF

HOW SUPPLIED

2 cc Mix-O-Vials; 500 mg

USUAL DOSE

1–3 cc

CAPSULE COMMENT

A cortisone product (similar to a hormone put out in stress by your own adrenal gland) that may be lifesaving in acute allergic reactions and any severe trauma or illness. A good case could be made for giving anyone you think was dying 3 cc of Solu-Cortef I.V. At the least it slows down the dying process and it may keep the patient going until he gets into a physician's care.

HOW IT WORKS

Solu-Cortef is a hormone similar to that put out by the adrenal glands, which helps the body respond to severe stress. It will help almost any dying patient because it delays response of destructive enzymes from the interior of dead or dying cells. Therefore, a case can be made for giving it to anyone who is dying of a catastrophic event such as a heart attack, auto accident, burn, or explosion. On the other hand, its use may be controversial, **so get from your responsible physician the specific indications he believes in.** One I.V. dose of 250 mg is not apt to hurt most people.

MOST AGREED UPON ADMINISTRATION

1. **After *adrenalin* has been given in anaphylaxis** or in acute **allergic reactions** such as occur after some insect bites. **Always give adrenalin *first!***
2. **Adrenal crisis.** If patient (usually a woman who has had surgery for breast cancer) has stopped taking cortisone and is in coma, an injection is worth giving.
3. Certain cases of severe asthma.
4. After all strokes, give 40 mg. I.V.
5. All drowning victims who may have water in lungs.

At any rate, keep it available. You will be surprised at how often a physician will tell you to use it if he knows you have it.

VALIUM

HOW SUPPLIED

10 mg
also available in prefilled syringes

USUAL DOSE

10 mg

CAPSULE COMMENT

Ten mg of Valium I.V. will harmlessly quiet most agitated patients and stop more convulsions. It has a wide safety margin.

XYLOCAINE (LIDOCAINE)

HOW SUPPLIED

5 cc ampules—20 mg per cc
75 mg prefilled syringe

USUAL DOSE

75 mg

CAPSULE COMMENT

The local anesthetic used by your dentist. It has become the *sine qua non* of cardiac arrhythmia treatment and has a wide range of safety. It acts as a local anesthetic to quiet an irritable heart (see pages 74–79).

USE

1. Use when EKG monitor shows **over six extra systoles per minute** (page 74).
2. Use after heart has been **converted** from **ventricular tachycardia** or **ventricular fibrillation** (pages 76 and 77).

HOW IT WORKS

This is the drug your dentist uses to "freeze" your jaw when he works. It acts the same way on the heart, i.e., it is a local anesthetic, which means it anesthetizes the heart muscle, which therefore does **not react** to stimuli (that ordinarily would make it beat) from an **abnormal focus** in the **ventricle**—which has been caused by acute heart damage.

1. Load with 75 mg I.V. in 10 seconds.
2. Drip in 75 mg in liter of Ringer's Lactate at rate to keep PVCs less than six/minute.

How to Buy an EKG Machine, an Electric Defibrillator

How to Use a Defibrillator

How to Recognize Basic EKG Patterns

What follows are the basics of EKG reading that the emergency personnel would know—and, in my opinion, is really **all** they have to know.

Once you have **mastered** this I am sure you **will want to know more** and, hopefully, ways will be found to teach you.

EKG MONITORS AND ELECTRICAL DEFIBRILLATORS

Many, many portable EKG monitors and defibrillators are available and the one you will choose should depend on local factors. A check list regarding important characteristics of dependability is as follows.

Buyer's Checklist—Choose the brand with the most yeses.

Characteristics	Brand A		Brand B		Brand C	
	Yes	No	Yes	No	Yes	No
1. Capable of 400 watt/sec						
2. Paddles at least 3 inch diameter						
3. Floating output						
4. Locking connector on paddle cable						
5. Self-discharge after turn-off						
6. Switch in handle of paddle						
7. Overcharge reduced by control knob						
8. Recharge time less than 10 seconds						
9. Circuit breaker or spare fuse						
10. Paddles easy to hold and apply						
11. Paddles designed for heavy duty use						
12. Can be synchronized for cardioversion						
13. Teaching sessions with machine						
14. Seller readily available for service						

A defibrillator, cardioscope, and **EKG** machine (battery operated) can be had for $3,000 at this writing. Many brands are available, and in that price range we suggest you choose the one in which the seller will teach you how to take good EKGs; will instruct you in the mechanics of applying electrical shock; will be available for good service; and will supply a loaner when yours is being adjusted.*

The main point is to practice on each other, taking EKGs until it is second nature. (If your group, when trained, has a monthly refresher meeting, let each person start with a **heart attack system** drill in which an EKG is taken.) The man who sells you the machine must agree to teach all of your group how to use it and make this clear to him before you buy it.

Usually the main difficulty is in getting a good initial connection to the chest. I suggest using the taped electrodes that are stuck to the chest (carry a razor to quickly get the hair off if necessary). I think also that a visual readout and a written readout capability are necessary. When you see something on the oscilliscope, you then can get a readout to use for your decision making.

Remember, listen to the heart **before** hookup of the EKG! If the heart has **stopped—external cardiac massage is the first priority** (page 120).

Do this: Have a bystander, if necessary, start **bag breathing** and let the #2 man hook up the EKG after he has started an I.V. At that point, **treatment is more important than diagnosis.**

Use of the Defibrillator

When it becomes necessary to **convert** a rhythm electrically, bare the chest, put on some conductor—water will do, set your **defibrillator** at 400 watt/sec, have everybody stand back, *disconnect* your EKG monitors, place the paddles on the chest, and push the buttons giving the patient the current. **Observe the rhythm obtained** for 60 seconds. If you have **not converted, try again** for at least **six times** at *2 minute intervals.*

*As soon as they are available get one that will deliver up to 1000 watt/sec. for fat people.

ON HOW TO RECOGNIZE FIVE IMPORTANT EKG PATTERNS THAT MAY HELP YOU SAVE A LIFE

A basic premise of SLS is that a reasonably intelligent individual can interpret an electrocardiogram (EKG) well enough to make decisions regarding changing a potentially dangerous rhythm of the heart to one that will give the patient a better chance of survival. The technique of *taking* EKGs should be taught you by the person who sells you the equipment.

One way of looking at EKG reading by SLS trainees is that, **if one can positively recognize five patterns,** he will have a fighting chance of saving most of the lives that are lost due to **rhythm problems** after a heart attack, and **rhythm problems** are the most common causes of death in heart attacks.

FIRST IMPORTANT PATTERN— *NORMAL SINUS RHYTHM*

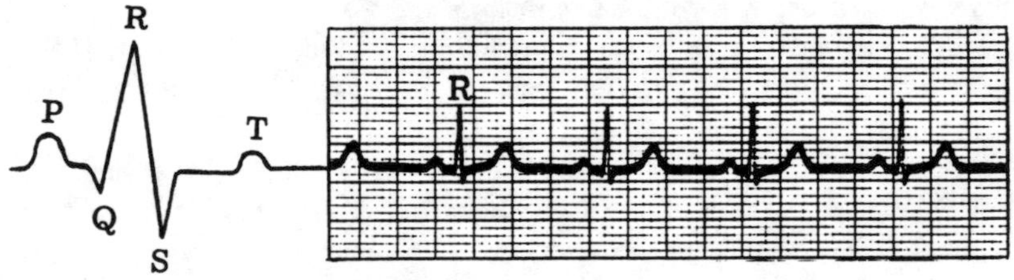

NORMAL RHYTHM

In **normal sinus rhythm** the *first* **upward** deflection is a **P wave**—it represents contraction of the top of the heart (the **auricle**). From the SLS point of view, **if you see a P wave—no matter what else you see, *this rules out* the need for electrical conversion!**

The *first* **downward** deflection is the **Q wave.**

The *second* **upward** deflection is the **R wave.**

The *second* **downward** deflection is the **S wave.**

The *third* **upward** deflection is the **T wave.**

The QRS waves form a complex, the shape of which you should fix in your mind. (Doodle complexes constantly for the next week after you read this.) You *must*—I repeat, ***must***—be able to decide if most of the major complexes you see are normal QRS complexes *or* complexes coming from the **bottom** of the heart—the **ventricle**. Ventricle complexes look different from the normal QRS complexes because they **do not have a P wave preceding them**, and they are usually **wider, higher,** and **less symmetrical** than a normal QRS complex. Practice distinguishing between normal QRS and ventricular complexes with your *flash cards* (pages 159–166) until you can tell at a glance.

THE SECOND IMPORTANT EKG PATTERN—VENTRICULAR EXTRA SYSTOLES

Once you have fixed the normal QRS complexes in your mind, your next **must** is to be able to recognize **ventricular extra systoles.**

This can be done by exclusion—**if the first deflection is not a P wave** and **if there is not a usual type of QRS complex** (and the QRS complex is remarkably constant in appearance)—**you are probably dealing with ventricular extra systoles.**

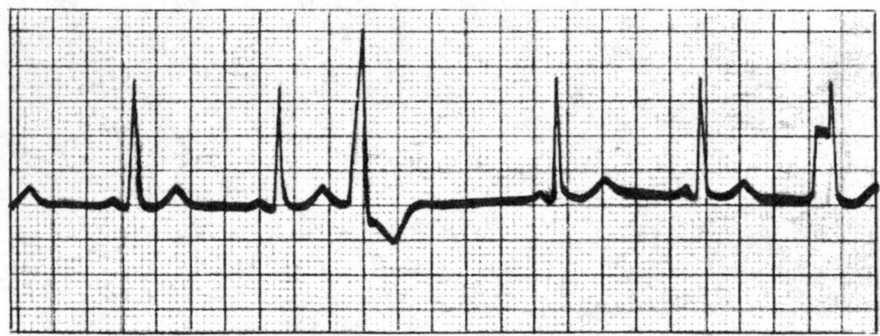

VENTRICULAR SYSTOLE

Ventricular extra systoles in an ambulance patient means the heart is getting irritable and may be going off on a fatal tangent. The **more frequently** ventricular extra systoles occur—the **more dangerous** it is for the patient.

Over six ventricular extra systoles per minute (coming within 48 squares of each other) indicates the patient should be treated with **Lidocaine** (see page 54).

As long as the **ventricular extra systoles** are mixed with normal QRS complexes you are only in an **"impending doom"** situation.

When they become the **only** rhythm—you have **ventricular tachycardia** (page 76).

THE THIRD IMPORTANT EKG PATTERN—VENTRICULAR TACHYCARDIA

In this rhythm all the impulses to beat are coming from the **bottom** of the heart and **death will follow** if the patient's heart **is not converted back to a rhythm that starts at the top** (the **auricle**).

The two things to note are:

1. All the major deflections **do not look like the usual QRS complexes.**
2. There are ***no*** **P waves.**

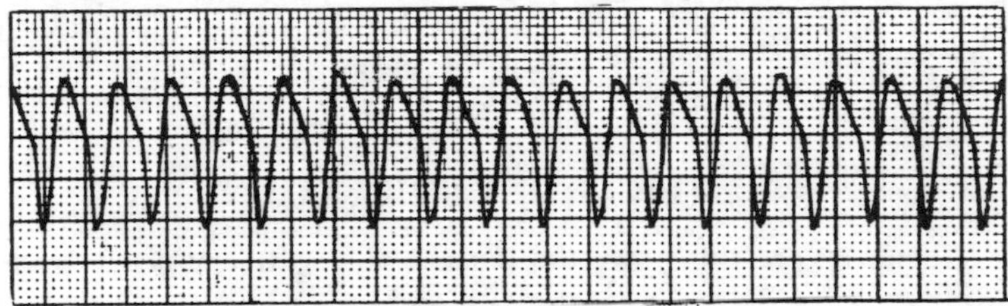

VENTRICULAR TACHYCARDIA

When you see this—give the patient 400 watt/sec of **electricity** with your **defibrillator** (page 57).

THE FOURTH IMPORTANT EKG PATTERN— VENTRICULAR FIBRILLATION

In this rhythm all impulses start *irregularly* from the bottom of the heart from various points in the **ventricle.** ***Death is imminent!*** The QRS complexes look even "crazier" than in **ventricular tachyardia,** and there **is no regular rhythm.**

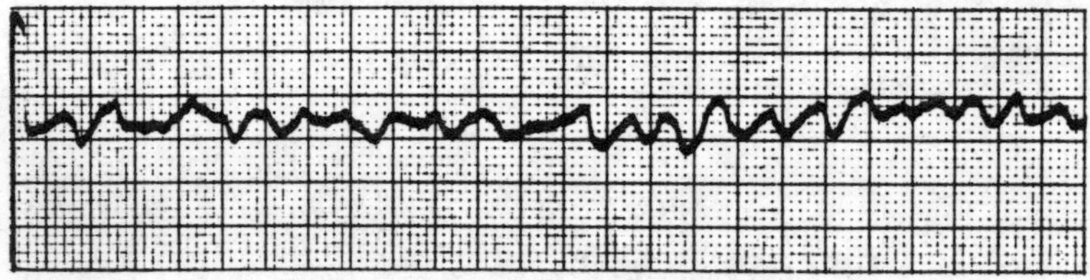

VENTRICULAR FIBRILLATION

When you see this—give the patient 400 watt/sec of **electricity** with your **defibrillator** for at **least 10 times** or **until you have converted the heart to some other rhythm** (page 57).

Continue **cardiac resuscitation massage** until rhythm reverts to something else or an adequate blood pressure returns.

THE FIFTH IMPORTANT EKG PATTERN—BRADYCARDIA

Bradycardia—the ***slow heart*** (see page 78). Often after a heart attack the heart becomes *very* **slow**.

A heart rate **below 60** usually is **dangerous** so, if the space between the complexes is **over five large squares, Atropine** is indicated—1/150 grain, subcutaneously, at the outer aspect of the arm.

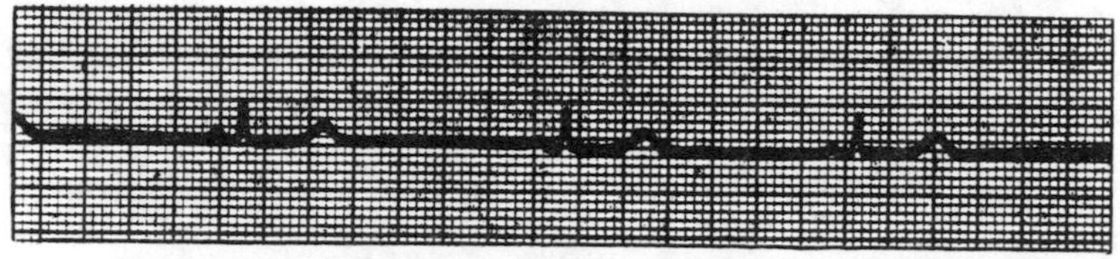

SINUS BRADYCARDIA

To measure your heart rate:

1. Put your **stethoscope** on the chest and count the beats for one full minute; **or**
2. Measure the space between the major complexes and use the chart on page 65.

An EKG other than—normal sinus, normal sinus with ventricular extra systoles, ventricular tachycardia, ventricular fibrillation, or bradycardia—requires no reaction on the simulated lifesaving level.*

The clues that tell you an EKG represents other than one of the five patterns mentioned above are **P waves**. These are waves representing contractions of the top of the heart (the **auricle**). When the heart is going **fast** they may be hard to find and separate from **T waves** (the last wave of the EKG) but if there are **two** deflections between the major deflections (QRS complex) and one of them is **upward, you can assume you have an auricular rhythm.**

This assumption allows you to relax from a Simulated Life Saving standpoint because, with an **auricular rhythm** and an **adequate blood pressure** (page 79, step 1), your patient will probably make it to the hospital.

*See page 79 for possible exception if decided upon by your Directing Physician.

TABLE TO DETERMINE APPROXIMATE HEART RATE ON EKG

NORMAL SINUS RHYTHM

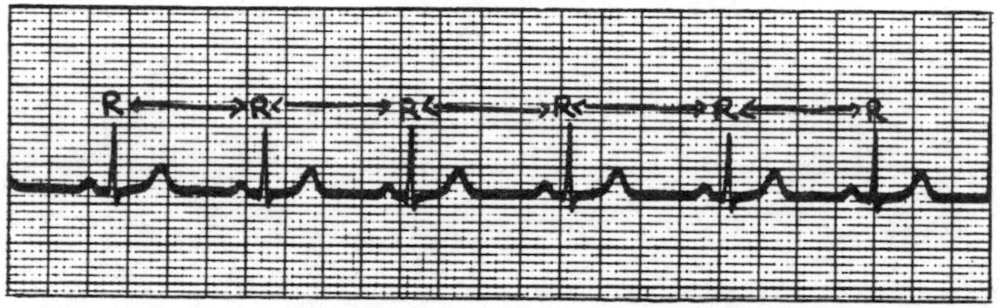

COUNT LARGE SQUARES BETWEEN R WAVES

Description of Rate	No. of Large Squares	Approximate Rate
Tachycardia*	Less than One	Over 300 beats/min
(Too fast)	Less than Two	Over 150 beats/min
	Less than Three	Over 100 beats/min
Normal Rate	Four or Five	Between 60 & 100 beats/min
Bradycardia	More than Five	Between 50 & 60 beats/min
(Too slow)	More than Six	Less than 50 beats/min

*If space between R waves is regular, P waves are present, and QRS pattern is normal, it is called Sinus Tachycardia.

NOTES

Simulated Lifesaving (S.L.S.) Systems and Emergency Care

Each system should be gone over carefully with your Directing Physician. The blank pages after each system are for the modifications that are decided upon between you.

NOTES

KNOW THE NEXT EIGHT PAGES COMPLETELY AND CHANCES ARE THAT YOU WILL SAVE A LIFE DURING YOUR OWN LIFETIME

Systems for When the Heart Stops

DIAGRAM OF STEPS USED TO START HEART

i.e. the material covered in pages 71–81

STEPS

1.
2.
3.
4.

} Assignment of jobs to each member of three-man team to the point when **heart is started— then—**

Step 5 and thereafter depend on EKG rhythm:

SYSTEMS FOR WHEN THE HEART STOPS—CARDIAC ARREST

The sudden stopping of the heart is usually due to the **shock** of the **heart attack** and you can sometimes get things going again by following this **system** exactly. Train yourselves to do this as a **three-man team.** If you have **only two men—enlist a passerby.** Instruct him in the **bag breathing** (page 11). With a **three-man team,** the steps to be presented each have three things to be done. Decide immediately who is to be **#1 man, #2 man,** and **#3 man.** The **leader is #1 man and he gives the orders.**

Step 1

#1 man—Listens to heart with **stethoscope.** If heart has **stopped,** he instructs **#2 man** to start **external cardiac massage*** and **#3 man** to start **bag breathing.**

#2 man—**External cardiac massage** at rate of 60/min—synchronized at five-to-one of **bag breathing.**

#3 man—Checks airway (page 11) and starts **bag breathing.**

Next—

Step 2

#1 man—

a. Brings O_2 to **bag breather.**
b. Gives 2 cc of **adrenalin** into the heart **in** and **upward** with a **spinal needle** (3 inches in) and 2 cc of **adrenalin I.V.** (page 32).
c. Hooks up EKG and starts recording so that everyone will know when the heart **starts** and **what rhythm it is in.**
d. He then starts the I.V. with Ringer's Lactate.
e. As soon as the I.V. has been started he injects three ampules of $NaHCO_3$ (soda bicarbonate).
f. He then places on the **blood pressure cuff** to see if the massage is giving any kind of blood pressure.

*To review the procedure for **external cardiac massage,** turn to page 120.

While he is doing this the other two men continue **external cardiac massage** and **bag breathing** until the heart starts **or** for 15 minutes (longer if the patient is young).

Step 3

As soon as the **heart stops** as indicated on the EKG, stop the massage and the **#2 man** can then take the **blood pressure**. If there is only electrical action and blood pressure is *under* 40, **go back to external massage for 3 minutes** while **cardiogenic shock system** (page 74, Step 8) is instituted.

Step 4

As soon as the **heart starts** take a one lead EKG and make a decision as to which of the following rhythms are most likely. Use pages 58 through 65.

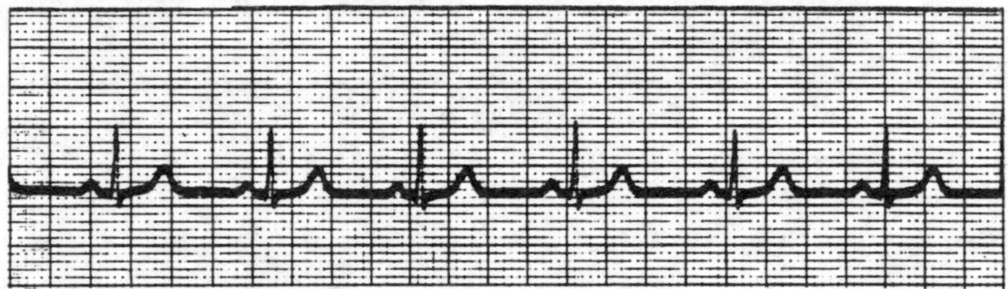

1. **Normal sinus rhythm**—if this, turn to page 74.

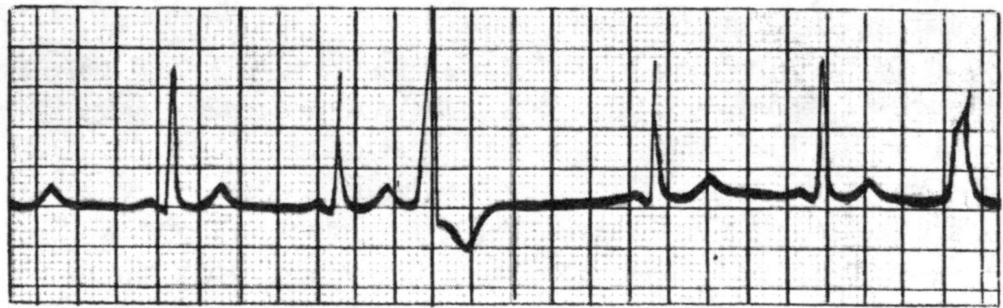

2. **Normal sinus rhythm** with **ventricular extra systoles**—if this, turn to page 75.

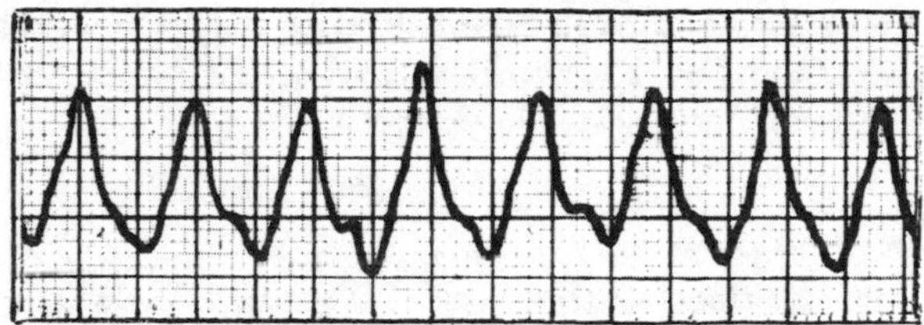

3. **Ventricular tachycardia**—if this, turn to page 76.

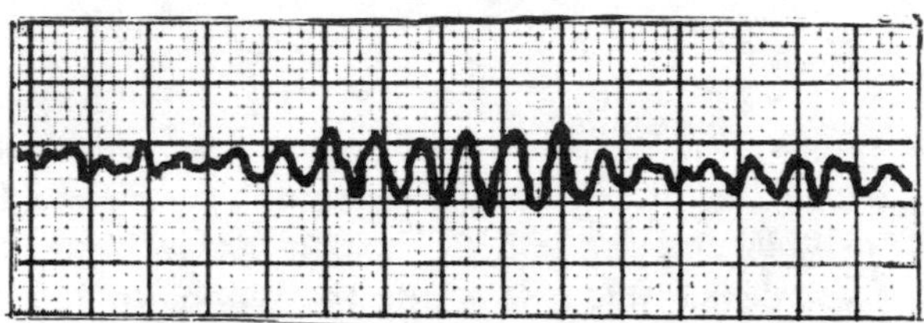

4. **Ventricular fibrillation**—if this, turn to page 77.

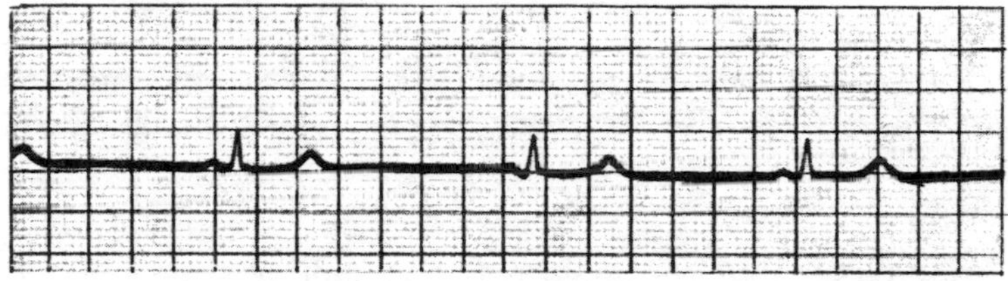

5. **Sinus bradycardia** (heart rate *under* 60)—if this, turn to page 78.
6. If **heart starts** with *any other rhythm* than (1) through (5), turn to page 79.

HEART STARTED WITH NORMAL SINUS RHYTHM AFTER CARDIOPULMONARY RESUSCITATION

Step 5

With **normal sinus** rhythm you will just have to watch for any **ventricular extra systoles** and, if they occur, give 2 cc of **Lidocaine,** 75 mg, into the I.V. tubing.

Step 6

If the rate is over 70 (*less* than 5 large squares between the R waves) (page 65) and blood pressure is over 90, put 500 mg (25 cc—five vials) of **Lidocaine** in the I.V. Lactated Ringer's bottle that is running. If you **cannot find a vein,** give the **Lidocaine,** ***100 mg,*** **into the muscle.** This is to prevent further arrhythmia.

Step 7

If the rate is under 60 (*more* than five large squares between the R waves) (page 65), give **Atropine,** one cc (gr 1/160) **into the muscle.**

Step 8

Now turn to the **blood pressure**. If the systolic pressure is *over* 90, your patient is ready for transport. If the blood pressure is *below* 90,* **add** 80 mg (2 cc) of **Dopamine** to the I.V. that is running at 40 drops/min (page 22). ***Always have Lidocaine n the I.V. with the Dopamine*** and be ready for rhythm changes. If they occur, turn to the appropriate pages during transport: **ventricular extra systoles** (page 75); **ventricular tachycardia** (page 76); **ventricular fibrillation** (page 77); or **sinus bradycardia** (page 78).

*We consider a blood pressure under 90 after a heart attack to mean **cardiogenic shock** and the Dopamine treats it. Your physician may want to go under 80 before the Dopamine.

HEART STARTS WITH NORMAL SINUS RHYTHM WITH VENTRICULAR EXTRA SYSTOLES

Step 5

With **normal sinus rhythm**, a rate over 60, and **ventricular extra systoles** give 75 mg **Lidocaine** (page 54) and put 500 mg (25 cc—five vials) in the I.V. bottle and run at 40 drops/min.

Step 6

If the rate is under 60 (*more* than five large squares between the R waves) (page 65) give **Atropine**, one cc (gr 1/160) into the muscle, or one cc I.V. if I.V. is running.

Step 7

Now turn to the **blood pressure.** If the systolic pressure is *over* 90, your patient is ready for transport. If the blood pressure is *below* 90,* **add** 80 mg (2 cc) of *Dopamine* to the I.V. that is running at 40 drops/min (page 22). ***Always have Lidocaine in the I.V. with the Dopamine*** and be ready for rhythm changes. If they occur, turn to the appropriate pages during transport: **ventricular tachycardia** (page 76); **ventricular fibrillation** (page 77); or **sinus bradycardia** (page 78).

*We consider a blood pressure under 90 after a heart attack to mean **cardiogenic shock** and the Dopamine treats it. Your physician may want to go under 80 before the Dopamine.

HEART STARTS WITH VENTRICULAR TACHYCARDIA

Step 5

At this point it will be necessary to **convert** this rhythm to something else with electricity, so bare the chest, put on some conductor—water will do, set your **defibrillator** at 400 watt/sec, have everybody stand back, *disconnect* your EKG monitors, place the paddles on the chest, and push the buttons giving the patient the current. **Observe the rhythm obtained** for 60 seconds. If you have **not converted, try again** for at least **six times** at *2-minute intervals.*

Step 6

If you cause **cardiac arrest**, again *start over* from page 70.

Step 7

Have **Lidocaine** running while you **convert**, 500 mg in the Lactated Ringer's that is running.

Step 8

If, after six times, you have **not converted**, transport the patient with his **ventricular tachycardia**—he may survive until seen by the physician. Continue to use CPR if systolic B.P. is *under 80.*

Step 9

With **normal sinus rhythm** you will just have to watch for any **ventricular extra systoles** and, if they occur, give 2 cc of **Lidocaine**, 5 mg, into the I.V. tubing.

Step 10

If the rate is under 60 (*more* than five large squares between the R waves) (page 65) give **Atropine,** one cc (gr 1/160) into the muscle.

Step 11

Now turn to the **blood pressure**. If the systolic pressure is *over* 90, your patient is ready for transport. If the blood pressure is *below* 90,* **add** 80 mg (2 cc) of **Dopamine** to the I.V. that is running at 40 drops/min (page 22). ***Always have Lidocaine in the I.V. with the Dopamine*** and be ready for rhythm changes. If they occur, turn to the appropriate pages during transport: **ventricular extra systoles** (page 75); **ventricular fibrillation** (page 77); or **sinus bradycardia** (page 78).

*We consider blood pressure under 90 after a heart attack to mean **cardiogenic shock** and the Dopamine treats it. Your physicians may want to go under 80 before the Dopamine.

HEART STARTS WITH VENTRICULAR FIBRILLATION

Step 5

Ventricular fibrillation—this rhythm cannot last long before the heart **stops again**, so it **must be converted electrically**. So, bare the chest, put on some conductor—water will do, set your **defibrillator** at 400 watt/sec, have everybody stand back, *disconnect* your EKG monitors, place the paddles on the patient's chest, and push the buttons giving the patient the current. **Observe the rhythm obtained** for 60 seconds. If you have **not converted, try again**, for at least **four times** at *2-minute intervals*.

Step 6

If you cause **cardiac arrest**, again *start over* from page 70.

Step 7

Give **Lidocaine** as soon as you **convert**, 500 mg in the Lactated Ringer's that is running.

Step 8

If, after four times, you have **not converted**, transport the patient in with his **ventricular fibrillation**, keeping up CPR—he may survive until seen by the physician.

Step 9

With **normal sinus rhythm** you will just have to watch for any **ventricular extra systoles** and, if they occur, give 3 cc of **Lidocaine**, 75 mg, into the I.V. tubing, then 3 mg per minute.

Step 10

If the rate is under 60 (*more* than five large squares between the R waves) (page 65) give **Atropine**, one cc (gr 1/160) **into the muscle.**

Step 11

Now turn to the **blood pressure**. If the systolic pressure is *over* 90, your patient is ready for transport. If the blood pressure is *below* 90,* **add** 80 mg (2 cc) of **Dopamine** to the I.V. that is running at 40 drops/min (page 22). ***Always have Lidocaine in the I.V. with the Dopamine***, and be ready for rhythm changes. If they occur, turn to the appropriate pages during transport: **ventricular extra systoles** (page 75); **ventricular tachycardia** (page 76); or **sinus bradycardia** (page 78).

*We consider a blood pressure under 90 after a heart attack to mean **cardiogenic shock** and the Dopamine treats it. Your physicians may want to go under 80 before the Dopamine.

HEART STARTS WITH SINUS BRADYCARDIA

Step 5

Give **Atropine**, 0.6–1.0 mg I.V. You may **repeat** in 30 minutes if heart rate **quickens initially** but then **slows again**.

Step 6

With **normal sinus rhythm** you will just have to watch for any **ventricular extra systoles** and, if they occur, give 3 cc of **Lidocaine**, 75 mg, into the I.V. tubing—then 3 mg/min.

Step 7

If the rate gets over 70 (*less* than five large squares between the R waves) (page 65), put 500 mg of **Lidocaine** in the I.V. Lactated Ringer's bottle that is running. If you **cannot find a vein** give the **Lidocaine**, 100 mg, **into the muscle.**

Step 8

If the rate is under 60 (*more* than five large squares between the R waves) (page 65) give **Atropine**, 0.6–1.0 mg I.V.

Step 9

Now turn to the **blood pressure**. If the systolic pressure is *over* 90, your patient is ready for transport. If the blood pressure is *below* 90,* **add** 80 mg (2 cc) of **Dopamine** to the I.V. that is running at 40 drops/min (page 22). ***Always have Lidocaine in the I.V. with the Dopamine*** and be ready for rhythm changes. If they occur, turn to the appropriate pages during transport: **ventricular extra systoles** (page 75); **ventricular tachycardia** (page 76); or **ventricular fibrillation** (page 77).

*We consider a blood pressure under 90 after a heart attack to mean **cardiogenic shock** and the Dopamine treats it. Your physicians may want to go under 80 before the Dopamine.

When the heart starts with any other rhythm than those on the preceding papers—follow this program—**providing you have been so directed.**

1. If the heart is going rapidly (over 120) but there is blood pressure and no pain, transport as is.
2. If the heart is going rapidly (over 200) or there is increasing chest pain, or systolic blood pressure under 85, use the following sequence.
   a. Carotid massage—right side for 10 seconds; if no slowing, go to *b*.
   b. Gag patient with tongue depressor two times while using carotid massage—if no slowing go to *c*.
   c. Tensilon 10 mg I.V.; if no slowing go to *d*.
   d. If patient comfortable, Inderal 1 mg I.V.: if no slowing go to *e*.
   e. Digoxin .5 mg I.V.; if in 3 minutes no slowing, repeat.
   f. If at this time patient is "going downhill" (i.e. looks like he is going to die) give another jolt of current first with 100 watt/sec, then with 200 and then with 300.

NOTES

NOTES AND MODIFICATIONS OF THE SYSTEM TO MANAGE A HEART THAT HAS STOPPED SUGGESTED BY YOUR DIRECTING PHYSICIAN

Note here his or her suggestions regarding: Dopamine, Digoxin, Tensilon, Lidocaine, intracardiac Adrenalin, and the use of $NaHCO_3$. Have him or her give you specific directions that he can give you written permission to use (depending of course on the political climate in the emergency medical field in your area at the time you receive instruction.)

SYSTEM FOR THE UNCONSCIOUS PATIENT

Coma

1. Listen to the heart with the stethoscope. If it has **stopped—start cardiopulmonary resuscitation system** (pages 120–121).
2. Note if patient is breathing—**if not, start bag breathing** (page 11).
3. Look for **bleeding.** If it is present, put *pressure* on it and go to the **hemorrhage system** (pages 18, 90, 102, 104).
4. Take **blood pressure** (page 10). If systolic is under 100, assume patient is in **shock** and start **shock system** (page 102).
5. Pay attention to **airway**. If the patient is breathing, tilt his head back and to the side and, if you **hear gurgling, clear back of throat with your finger and/or the suction machine.**
6. Now consider **drug overdose**. If there are needle marks or other reasons to consider drug usage—such as syringe in room itself—**give** .4 mg Narcan into the vein (page 46). If the patient wakes up suddenly, **you have saved a life.**
7. Do a **finger prick blood sugar** and if distinct **elevation** (over 250), start **diabetic coma system** (page 84). If the blood sugar is under 70—give 50 cc of 50% glucose, repeating if the patient comes to and then lapses again into coma (**insulin reaction system,** page 116).

At this point you have done all you probably can do to help at the spot, so **transport** carefully.

Bring along any medicine bottles or pills that may be lying around. Try to find out what happened and note this information in your report (page 132).

Diagnoses at this point, are, in order of likelihood: **stroke, acute alcoholism, drug overdose,** or **kidney failure with uremia.**

Always follow up these patients so you know what the **diagnosis** really was.

Suggestions of Directing Physicians regarding the unconscious patient.

DIABETIC COMA SYSTEM

You will arrive at this diagnosis through your **unconscious patient system** (page 82), when your blood sugar stick shows over 250 mg% of sugar. In addition, patients with **diabetic coma** also breathe very deeply and rapidly and their skin is very dry.

1. Look to *airway* and see that there is free access to air.
2. Keep patient warm and bundle securely.
3. Start Lactated Ringer's I.V. and run at 100 drops/min.
4. **This is only if your Directing Physician agrees:**
   a. Give 50 units of regular insulin I.V. (page 44). **Do not give** unless blood sugar is over 250.
   b. Give three ampules of $NaHCO_3$ (**sodabicarb**) (page 51).
5. Transport.

NOTE

Some cases of **stroke** will be unconscious and have an elevated blood sugar so—**if there is paralysis of one side, use stroke system.**

AGREED UPON MODIFICATIONS OF THE DIABETIC COMA SYSTEM

1. How much and by what route does your physician want you to give **insulin**?
2. Some physicians would like some $NaHCO_3$ (sodabicarbonate) given to these patients. Get an opinion regarding this.

SYSTEM FOR HEART ATTACK OR SEVERE CHEST PAIN

Assume that any patient complaining of a **severe chest pain has had a heart attack**!

1. **Reassure him**—tell him that "the marines have landed, everything is under control."*
2. Keep him **sitting up** and **loosen his collar**.
3. **Listen to his heart** and **take his blood pressure**.
4. **Take an EKG:**

   If he does ***not*** **have ventricular systoles**—

   If he does—turn to page 75.

   And if he does ***not*** **have ventricular tachycardia**—

   If he does—turn to page 76.

   And if he does ***not*** **have ventricular fibrillation**—

   If he does—turn to page 77.

   And if his **blood pressue is over 90**—

   If under 100—turn to page 74, Step 8.

   And if his **rate is between 60 and 200** (page 65).

   If his **rate is greater than 200 or less than 60**—turn to pages 78 or 79.
5. **Start** him on oxygen by mask or nasal catheter, 6 liters/min, and transport him under monitor—**sitting up**.
6. **Stay with him** in the Emergency Room until you have given your report (page 132) and the EKG strips to the *responsible person* in the Admitting Room. I would even get a receipt for him so that the Admitting Room person realizes the responsibility is now his.

   This simple procedure is the best for the majority of heart attacks.

*If you are set up to give **Morphine**, give gr 1/4 with 1/150 gr of **Atropine** (page 35).

MODIFICATIONS BY YOUR DIRECTING PHYSICIAN FOR THE HEART ATTACK SYSTEM

SYSTEM FOR MANAGEMENT OF CONGESTIVE HEART FAILURE

The type of patient you can help in **congestive heart failure** is relatively easy to recognize.

If the patient

—Is over 60
—Is a known cardiac
—Has a pulse rate over 100
—Is very short of breath
—Is bluish in appearance
—Has been on digitalis in the past
—Seems to have increasing difficulty in breathing
—Has bulging neck veins

Do the following

—Start O_2 while reassuring the patient.
—Keep him sitting up.
—Put **tourniquets** on *three* of his four limbs, *alternately*, for 10 minutes. (Practice this with your Directing Physician.) This will ***decrease*** the amount of blood returning to the heart and **decrease lung congestion.**

On prior permission or voice contact with your Directing Physician:
Give 40 mg **Lasix I.V.** (page 45)
Give Morphine, 7 mg I.M.

MODIFICATIONS BY YOUR DIRECTING PHYSICIAN FOR THE CONGESTIVE HEART FAILURE SYSTEM

Get a directive from your Directing Physician regarding **Digoxin**.

If you are sure the patient has never had **Digitalis** in the past, some physicians (including myself) would like you to give it. Others will be against the idea.

SHOCK SYSTEM FOR PATIENT WHO IS SICK AND HAS A SYSTOLIC BLOOD PRESSURE UNDER 90

Shock is a condition caused by not enough blood with oxygen in it reaching the body's cells. It might be considered the first phase of dying. It is more easily **prevented than treated.**

Prevention of Shock

In any seriously ill or injured patient:

1. Keep patient warm and reassure him vigorously
2. Have patient lying down so as to have gravity help get blood to his brain.
3. Start an I.V. with Lactated Ringer's on any seriously injured patient. Have it run at 84 drops per minute.

Treatment of Shock

1. Diagnose **shock** with your eyes and the **blood pressure cuff.** The patient will be cold, clammy, and often sweating. His pulse will be rapid and his **systolic blood pressure will be below 90.**
2. Cover him with several blankets and have him lying down.
3. Start I.V. with Lactated Ringer's at 150 drops per minute and take his **blood pressure often**—decrease rate of I.V. when blood pressure rises to 100.

4. **Try to decide cause of shock.** In order of probability these are:

Heart attack (page 86) **Bleeding ulcer** (page 102) **Bleeding elsewhere** (page 104) **Severe traumatic injury** (page 97) **Burn shock** (page 107)	Decide on which you think is most probable and turn to page indicated. It is doubtful that you could harm a patient even if you make a wrong guess.

Follow directions on appropriate pages.

5. **This is only if your Directing Physician agrees:** If the blood pressure is **below 50** and you have a definite idea of what is causing the **shock—add** 2 cc of Dopamine to the I.V. Lactated Ringer's and let it flow at rate to get blood pressure to 90. (This **may** speed up the heart too much. If it goes to a rate of over 150/min, you may have to settle for a little slower rate.) ***If there is blood loss shock—do not do this!***
6. Hook up the EKG and monitor the heart, treating **ventricular rhythms** as they occur (pages 60, 61, 62).

AGREED UPON MODIFICATIONS OF SHOCK SYSTEM

SYSTEM FOR STROKE OR BRAIN HEMORRHAGE

The patient's family will usually tell you right away that he had a **stroke** and they probably will be right. At any rate, when an older person becomes paralyzed in an arm or leg, or suddenly cannot speak, he probably has had a **stroke** and should be treated for such.

1. Keep head slightly **elevated** and **to the side**.
2. Check **airway** and use **suction machine** if necessary.
3. Check **blood pressure** and **listen to the heart**. If the **blood pressure** is **over 100** systolic and the **heart rate** is over 60—**bring the patient in.**
4. Give 8 mg of Decadron I.V. to reduce brain swelling and hopefully to preserve function.

Watch for sudden vomiting and **aspiration!** (Have your **suction machine** ready.)

Include in your report (page 132) as much information as you can regarding past medication, recent blows on the head, and whether or not the patient has had high blood pressure in the past.

AGREED UPON MODIFICATIONS OF STROKE SYSTEM

SYSTEM FOR DRUG OVERDOSE

If you have reason to believe an unconscious patient is a hard drug addict, or **if there is even a faint suspicion of it—give:**

1. Narcan 2 cc I.V. (8 mg) **immediately.** If he wakes up you were right (page 46).
2. Even while the Narcan is being given—**start ventilation with the bag if the respirations are *under* 12, since most drug overdoses die of breathing failure. Add 100% oxygen and keep up continuous artificial respiration.**
3. Start an I.V. with Lactated Ringer's at 84 drops per minute. (This will help wash out most other drugs from the system.)
4. Collect urine if possible and give this to the Admitting Ward personnel, since it can be tested immediately for which drug caused the difficulty.
5. Get as much history as you can, and take in any bottles, pills, or capsules that may be around. (**Do *not* put into writing any suspicion you have regarding addiction, however, since it can be used against you if you are wrong.**)

AGREED UPON MODIFICATIONS OF DRUG OVERDOSE SYSTEM

AUTO ACCIDENT SYSTEM

The **first** consideration in auto accidents is what is called **triage,** which simply means—**decide on the order in which the patient should be treated.**

Considerations in order of importance:

I. Airway

If a patient is obviously dying because the throat is crushed or the face is bashed in so that he cannot get air into his lungs—**establish an airway by:**

1. Scooping out mouth and throat area with your finger.
2. Aspirating (Airway equipment—page 11).
3. Trying a pharyngeal airway.
   If he is still choking to death try:
4. An **endotracheal tube** (page 13); **or** Put the **#14 needle** below the Adam's apple (page 15).

   But only if your Directing Physician has given you the go ahead!

II. Hemorrhage

Use **Hemorrhage System** (pages 18, 102)

III. Shock

All seriously injured patients are to be treated for shock!

1. **Prevent shock** by keeping patient warm.
2. Start Lactated Ringer's I.V. (84 drops per minute).

Only by order of physician

3. Give morphine to patients in severe pain—**if** they have **no breathing problems.**
4. **Spinal injuries**—splint as you have been taught in your EMT* course. (Hopefully, by the time this manual appears, you will be able then to call for a helicopter for the transport of the patient to a Spinal Injury Center.)

*Emergency Medical Technician's Course

5. **Fractures**—splint as per your EMT course. Treat **compound fracture** as you would any other wound, i.e., a sterile dressing and a bandage.
6. **Crushed chest**—see **Chest Injury System** (page 100).
7. Gather all medical information of the patient's past history that you can and include it in the Data list of your report.

AGREED UPON MODIFICATIONS FOR AUTO ACCIDENTS

Treatment of spinal injuries and head injuries depend on local facilities and helicopter transport—so work out the best system for your area.

CHEST INJURY SYSTEM

Two conditions come to mind in which lives might be saved by emergency care of a **chest injury**.

1. **Tension pneumothorax**—In this situation the patient sucks in air through a wound in the chest wall and the air cannot get out. This trapped air forces the lung to collapse. Therefore, when a patient has a chest wound (steering wheel is the most common cause) and is having increasing shortness of breath (he may be turning blue), place the valved # 14 needle from your Jump Kit below the middle of the clavicle (page 24). Put it in 2 inches or until you hear air escaping. Tape it in place. When inserting it point inward and downward. If you get pure blood back no real harm will have been done—merely draw it out and point it in at a slightly more downward angle.
2. When there are multiple **rib fractures** or a **crushed sternum**, the rib cage may not be stable enough for inhaling. In this situation:
   Place on side to stabilize one-half of the rib cage.
   Bag breathe the patient.
   Morphine will be very helpful here—**but only if authorized by your Directing Physician.**

AGREED UPON MODIFICATIONS OF CHEST INJURY SYSTEM

Discuss thoroughly with your Directing Physician his feelings about the crushed chest and endotracheal tubes (pages 12–14) used with **Morphine** and **bag breathing** (page 11). He may want you to handle them using these methods.

SYSTEM FOR GASTROINTESTINAL TRACT BLEEDING

Any acutely ill patient with:

1. Blood pressure **under 100**
2. Pulse **over 110**
3. A history of high **alcoholic** intake and/or an **ulcer** or **high aspirin** intake
4. **No** chest pain
5. Black, tarry—or even bloody—stools

may have a bleeding ulcer and be going into *blood loss shock.*

Therefore, start an I.V. with Lactated Ringer's at 100 drops per minute and call in ahead that you may be bringing in an **acute bleeding ulcer.**

Try to get history of **aspirin** or other medication intake.

AGREED UPON MODIFICATION OF BLEEDING ULCER SYSTEM

SYSTEM FOR A WOMAN IN LABOR OR BLEEDING FROM THE VAGINA*

1. Unless there are **unusual** aspects, transport the woman to the hospital in whatever position she finds most comfortable—usually lying down.
2. If she is having **severe hemorrhage**, that is, if there is much blood coming out from between her legs, or if she appears to have **fainted** or is in **shock**, start an I.V. with Lactated Ringer's and keep it running at 100 drops/min. Record blood pressure frequently. Call ahead to the hospital to report the situation since they may want her to go directly to the Operating Room. See page 43 regarding the use of **Ergotrate**.
3. Women show that they are in **labor** in three ways: **bleeding, contractions (labor pains),** or **leaking fluid from the bag of waters.**
   a. If the patient is **bleeding,** treat her as above (#2).
   b. If there is **leaking of fluid**, simply have the patient lying down and transport her to the hospital as soon as possible.
   c. If the patient is having **contractions** (**labor pains**), transport her to the hospital as soon as possible, particularly if the pains are **less than 10 minutes apart**.
   d. If the baby's head starts to come out of the vagina, **do the following**: Remove all undergarments. Spread sterile towels or sheets (or newspapers) beneath the buttocks and between the patient's legs. Do **not** do anything to hold back the head. Allow the woman to push if she feels the desire to do so. Let the baby's head come out by itself; then encourage the woman to push the shoulders out. Tie the umbilical cord in **two** places, approximately 8 inches from the baby's navel. (Use heavy cord or a strip of cloth.) Cut between those two ties. Use the obstetrical kit in your first aid kit for this (page 19).

*Prepared by Dr. Carl J. Levinson, Chief, Department of Obstetrics & Gynecology, Mount Sinai Medical Center, Milwaukee.

4. ***The baby.*** Wrap the baby in warm clothes, towels, etc. (It is **important to keep the child warm.**) Use a bulb syringe to clean out the baby's mouth and throat. **Be gentle. Make sure** the *cord is not bleeding*!
5. ***The afterbirth.*** The afterbirth will generally deliver by itself within five minutes after the delivery of the child. **Do not pull on the cord.** Once the afterbirth is in the vagina the mother will have an urge to push—encourage her to do so. Save the afterbirth in a metal or plastic container. If there is continued **bleeding,** treat as in #2 above. If there is evidence of **shock** or continued bleeding, be sure that the Lactated Ringer's I.V. is running at 60 to 80 drops per minute and give 2 cc of **Ergotrate** (page 43) to contract the uterus.

AGREED UPON MODIFICATION OF THE SYSTEM FOR A WOMAN IN LABOR OR BLEEDING FROM THE VAGINA

What is your Directing Physician's opinion about **Ergotrate**?

SYSTEM FOR BURN MANAGEMENT

1. The **most important thing to do for a severely burned patient** is to put in an I.V. and start Lactated Ringer's at 168 drops per minute—100 drops per minute if the patient is over 60 years of age.
2. Place a moistened sheet over his burned area.
3. ***Do not* put any ointments or medication** over his burned area.
4. Start the patient on **oxygen** by catheter at 6 liters per minute.
5. Usually there is not much pain, so **do not** give morphine unless there are other painful injuries—**and then only if authorized by your Directing Physician.**
6. Pay special attention to **airway** and **bag breathing** if necessary (pages 11–14).
7. **If agreed to by your Directing Physician** give Solu-Cortef to patients who have had an obvious pulmonary burn or who have inhaled a lot of smoke.

AGREED UPON MODIFICATION OF SYSTEM OF BURN MANAGEMENT

SYSTEM FOR LUNG FAILURE

A patient whose main complaint is that he cannot get air and **who is in acute distress** qualifies for the following System:

1. a. If the patient is a **known asthmatic—**
   b. Is under 55 years of age—
   c. Has responded to **adrenalin** before—
   —Give him 1 cc of **Adrenalin**, subcutaneously (page 32). This will usually give him immediate relief.
   d. If there is **no response** to the **adrenalin** and **if your Directing Physician has agreed—**
   —Give him Solu-Cortef (page 52).
2. If the patient has **no** history of asthma but if his breathing problem is essentially **wheezing** (you ought to be able to recognize a wheeze when you hear it), he may be having an acute **allergic reaction** (common after eating seafood, getting an antibiotic, being exposed to an aerosol can to which there is an allergy, or being stung by an insect).
   —Give him 1 cc of **adrenalin** (page 32) subcutaneously. If there is **no response to the adrenalin** and **if your Directing Physician has agreed—**give him Solu-Cortef (page 52).
3. Chronic emphysema patients, or those with severe chronic bronchitis, often will go into **respiratory distress** state. **Oxygen** itself is **poor** for these people because they are often breathing only because of the stimulus of oxygen lack. Therefore, if an older person, who is known to you as a respiratory problem, seems in acute distress—**give him oxygen only via bag breathing.**

Furthermore, do **not leave him in the Admitting Ward without bag breathing** until a responsible person has been apprised of the situation because, when you start to **bag breathe** him, **he may no longer be able to breathe by himself.**

So, be as sure as you can in your own mind **before you start to bag breathe a respiratory cripple**, that he **really needs it.**

The rule of thumb should be: **If he looks to you as if *he will die without oxygen*,** give it to him via **bag breathing.**

If he looks like he *might* make it *without* oxygen, you can try *bag breathing* him with *room air first.*

AGREED UPON MODIFICATION OF THE SYSTEM FOR BREATHING FAILURE AND/OR ASTHMA

There is much difference of opinion in this field and your Directing Physician may want to modify this System quite a bit.

SYSTEM FOR CARBON MONOXIDE POISONING

These are usually suicides or "neckers" in a closed car.

1. **Be careful** yourselves as you get them out—**carbon monoxide is odorless.**
2. Start O_2 by **bag breathing** immediately (page 11).
3. Transport to the nearest facility with a **hyperbaric oxygen** setup. These will all take direct admission of severe **carbon monoxide poisonings** because this is the prime indication for **hyperbaric oxygen** at the present time;

   or

   If **hyperbaric oxygen** is not available within 40 miles, or a helicopter is not on call, take to your regular hospital.
4. During transit, start an I.V. with Lactated Ringer's at 40 drops per minute if the patient is unconscious.

AGREED UPON MODIFICATION OF THE SYSTEM FOR CARBON MONOXIDE TREATMENT

SYSTEM FOR EMERGENCY CARE FOR EYES*

Immobilization of a **lacerated**, or **ruptured**, or badly **contused eye** is as important as splinting a fractured limb. This is accomplished by **patching both eyes.**

I. Injuries Causing Lacerations or Severe Contusions to the Eyeball

1. Patch both eyes with eye pads or gauze squares.
2. Keep patient lying quietly on back.
3. Administer medication for pain.
4. Do **not** place any medications in the eye.

II. Chemical Injuries to Eyeball

1. Irrigate eye with room temperature, or lukewarm, sterile eye or normal saline irrigating solution. (If sterile solution is not available, use plain tap water.)
2. Continue for *at least* 20 to 30 minutes.
3. If topical anesthetic is available, use 2 or 3 drops first.
4. Use lid retractor to hold lids open for better irrigation.
5. If particles of chemical matter can be seen in the eye, use 2 or 3 drops of topical anesthetic, and attempt to remove with a cotton swab or forceps.
6. Apply eye patch.
7. Give pain medication.

III. Thermal Burn to Eyeball

1. Apply sterile topical anesthetic if available.
2. Give pain medication.
3. Apply eye patch.
4. If particles in the eye, such as molten metal, give drops of topical anesthetic, and try to remove these with cotton swabs or forceps.
5. If lids are burned, apply antibiotic ointment.
6. If lid closure is impaired, apply antibiotic ointment to eye and apply patch.

*These pages were prepared by Herbert Giller, M.D., Ophthalmologist, Associate Clinical Professor of Ophthalmology of the Medical College of Wisconsin.

IV. Lid Lacerations

1. Stop active bleeding by applying mild pressure, but use care, since eyeball may be injured.
2. Apply sterile dressing.

V. Facial Fractures Involving Orbit

1. Keep patient quiet on back.
2. Be certain *adequate airway is maintained.*

VI. Corneal Abrasions

1. If the abrasion can be seen, then instill 1 or 2 drops of topical anesthetic (0.5% Tetracaine, e.g. pontocaine, or 0.5% Proparacaine, e.g. ophthaine) for relief of pain and patch the eye. ****Do not** instill topical anesthetics more than twice and never give topical anesthetic to the patient for home use.
2. Use systemic analgesics if needed.

VII. Superficial Foreign Bodies

1. Instill 1 or 2 drops of topical anesthetic as for corneal abrasion.
2. For conjunctival foreign body, moisten a cotton applicator with topical anesthetic and gently wipe away foreign body.**If cornea is scratched in vertical manner, foreign body may be under upper lid.
3. If foreign body is on the cornea, instill topical anesthetic; then attempt to dislodge it with a sterile hypodermic needle. **If it does not dislodge easily, leave it for the doctor.
4. Patch the eye.

AGREED UPON MODIFICATION OF THE SYSTEM FOR EMERGENCY CARE OF THE EYES

INSULIN REACTION SYSTEM

When a diabetic—**feels cold** and **clammy**
—is weak
—is on insulin
—sweats profusely
—even, occasionally, becomes violent

He may be suffering an *insulin reaction*!

If he is **conscious**—give him a piece of candy, a Coke, a sugar cube, orange juice—anything **sweet**. He usually becomes normal within 5 minutes.

When a **coma** patient has a **blood sugar below 70** on the finger prick stick (page 23), he **may** or **may not** be **cold** and **clammy** and **sweating**. Give him two ampules of **50% Glucose I.V.**—directly or into the tubing of an I.V. that has Lactated Ringer's running. If he was having an **insulin reaction**, he will usually wake up and can often be taken home.

An alternate method which probably is better than the use of 50% Glucose is the injection of Glucagon, 1 cc I.M., immediately and in 15 minutes. This is a natural hormone that increases blood sugar physiologically.

MODIFICATIONS BY YOUR DIRECTING PHYSICIAN OF THE INSULIN REACTION SYSTEM

SYSTEM FOR AN ACUTE ALLERGIC REACTION

When a person **collapses** and is in **acute distress following:**
—**A penicillin injection** (up to 2 hours)
—**An antibiotic taken by mouth**
—**A bee sting**
—**An aspirin**
—**Eating seafood**
—**Taking some medicine by mouth**

His life can often be saved if he is ***immediately*** given 1 cc of **adrenalin** subcutaneously (page 32) *and* 1 cc of **adrenalin** intravenously (page 32). Follow this with Solu-Cortef (page 52).

Start **bag breathing** him with oxygen at the same time and transport him.

If he is turning **blue** and **cannot get air** (caused by a spasm of his vocal cord box) either put down an **endotracheal tube** (page 13) or insert a **#14 gage needle** below the Adam's apple and hook up oxygen to it.

MODIFICATIONS BY THE DIRECTING PHYSICIAN OF THE ACUTE ALLERGIC REACTION SYSTEM

SYSTEM FOR EXTERNAL CARDIAC MASSAGE

1. If the heart has **stopped** as indicated either by no sound through your **stethoscope** or by a flat EKG—***external cardiac massage*** is the *first priority*! (Check airway quickly.)
2. Tell someone to get a board to place under the patient's back or lay him on the floor.
3. Kneel on either side of the patient and place the heel of your hand at the midpoint between, and just below, the nipples.
4. Place the heel of the other hand over the back of the hand on the chest and apply 80–120 pounds of pressure (enough to move the front of the chest down one inch) at 60 times per minute.
5. This is the **main priority** and *must be continued* at least until the pupils dilate completely—or maybe longer—or until the EKG shows the heart is beating.
6. If you happen to be alone, **stop** after every 15 heart compressions and do *two* mouth-to-mouth respirations (page 121).

Practice **external cardiac massage** on each other and on mannequins. Each person over the age of 12 should know how to do this. See that it is taught in your Junior High Schools, Boy Scout and Girl Scout Troops. Be sure your own children know this. They might save your life or that of your wife some day with it.

SYSTEM FOR MOUTH-TO-MOUTH RESPIRATION

1. If you do not have a bag, valve, mask device (page 11) for ventilation, **mouth-to-mouth** *must be done* if the patient is not breathing. Be sure to pinch the nostrils closed.
2. **External cardiac massage** must be going on at the same time if the heart has stopped.
3. Be *sure* the **airway** is clear by "hooking" the back of the throat with your finger.
4. Tilt the head back as far as you can by placing your fingers under the chin and your thumbs alongside the temples. Have somebody roll up a jacket or towel to put under the neck so that the head stays overextended.
5. Hold the nose of the patient, take a deep breath, open the patient's mouth, and blow into his mouth with enough force to expand his lungs. Do this 15 times per minute.
6. There are devices to put into patients' mouths for mouth-to-mouth breathing but we suggest you get a bag, valve, mask device rather than one of these and save mouth-to-mouth for times you are without your Jump Kit.
7. When the patient gasps, stop for a moment to see whether or not he may be starting to resume breathing on his own. If he is **not, resume the mouth-to-mouth**.
8. **Continue** at least as long as the pupils do not completely dilate—and perhaps longer.
9. With a baby you might have to cover the mouth and nose with your mouth.

Practice mouth-to-mouth on a mannequin, with a gauge that tells you how much pressure is necessary.

Be sure your entire family knows mouth-to-mouth resuscitation and discuss both this and **external cardiac massage** as a family unit. Every citizen over the age of 12 should know how to do this. See that it is taught in your Junior High Schools, High Schools, Boy Scout and Girl Scout Troops. Be sure your own children know this. They might save your life or that of your wife some day with it.

SYSTEM FOR DROWNING

Drowning victims may die suddenly for no apparent reason several hours after they are pulled from the water. Therefore when someone is rescued he should always be transported to an emergency room. His breathing and heart should be attended to by the usual methods (see CPR instructions on pages 120-121) but after this the following rules should be followed on all near victims who were actually immersed and in bona fide trouble.

1. Start an I.V. and give Solu-Cortef (page 52). This helps prevent unexplained pulmonary edema and cannot hurt the patient.
2. If patient was in *salt water*, start an I.V. at 200 cc per hour with 5% dextrose in water and give 60 mg of Lasix I.V. This will work out the salt in the blood and prevent damage it can cause.
3. If the patient was in *fresh water*, start an I.V. of Ringer's Lactate at 100 cc per hour and give 60 mg of Lasix I.V. to get rid of the water that dilutes the blood to the detriment of the patient.
4. Encourage the emergency room to get serial chest x-rays and blood gases for at least 8 hours after the incident.

SUGGESTIONS OF DIRECTING PHYSICIAN REGARDING DROWNING

SYSTEM FOR INITIAL CARE OF SPINAL INJURY

Automobile accidents provide half the fractured spines in the United States and half of these victims end up as paraplegics, so this dread injury must be thought of at the site of any serious automobile accident. The football field, swimming pool, and the trampoline all add additional victims.

The System is simple: **when there is any question of a spinal cord injury**, transport on a frame (page 20). We illustrate only one kind, but every emergency vehicle must have a device that will immobilize the entire spine.

Symptoms that suggest possibility of spine injury are:

1. Paralysis of any extremity;
2. Extreme pain in the neck or back on movement;
3. Pain shooting down on extremity on movement;
4. Inability to void after back trauma (often due to a compression fracture of the spine).

SUGGESTIONS OF DIRECTING PHYSICIAN REGARDING SPINAL INJURY

SYSTEM FOR SEVERE HEAD INJURY

Any injury that knocks a patient unconscious must be considered a serious, life-threatening head injury—at a minimum, the next 24 hours should be spent in bed under observation (not necessarily in the hospital).

1. Obtain a complete history:
   Direction of blow?
   Period of unconsciousness?
   Previous history of alcohol or drug ingestion?
   History of epilepsy?
   Did something that happened just before cause the patient to fall and hit his head?
   Things like coronaries and strokes must be considered.
   Sometimes you will find a bullet hole that is very inconspicuous.
2. Attend to airway and circulation. Shock and hypotension are relatively rare in "pure" head injuries, so if they are present, look for other causes.
3. Increasing yawning or hiccuping are danger signs that should get you going in regard to getting the patient to a neurosurgeon for decompression. Slowing of pulse has similar implications.
4. Examine and describe exactly the size of each pupil.
5. Look at base of skull and ears for clear fluid. This is spinal fluid leaking out and means you have a basal skull fracture.
6. If the pulse is slowing, the pupils enlarging, and the patient sinking deeper into unconsciousness, give Solu-Cortef (page 52) to reduce cerebral edema (get O.K. for this from your Directing Physician).

SUGGESTIONS OF DIRECTING PHYSICIAN REGARDING SEVERE HEAD INJURY

GENERAL RULES FOR THE TRAUMA VICTIM

At the scene of an accident where there might be multiple injuries and multiple patients, check over these points after you have attended to the obvious problems.

1. Splint all fractures—and treat patients for shock: warm blankets and reassurance—major bones—Demerol or Morphine.
2. Crush injuries even apparently minor should be treated for shock also. In addition, get good histories of how it happened and put it in your report. This may help reconstruction and tell eventual surgeons how much exploration they must do.
3. Be sure parents are informed that children with muscular skeletal injuries that hurt for more than a few days must be seen by a physician, as persisting symptoms usually mean serious undetected injury. Elbows in particular need consultation by an orthopedic surgeon if symptoms persist.
4. All cases of head injury should be taken seriously and patients transported to an emergency room for observation. Be sure they are accompanied even though ambulatory.
5. Dislocated shoulders are easy to diagnose and during the first half hour are relatively easy to snap into place by having the patient lie down, placing your left heel in the axilla and gently pulling the wrist toward you while externally rotating it (Figure 5).
6. Remember face injuries are rarely an emergency if airway is open and bleeding is not frank hemorrhage, so transport to place where specialty care is available if desirable. Serious lacerations and avulsive injuries are best handled by plastic surgeons and serious eye injuries by ophthalmologists, and rarely does definitive treatment have to be done before they arrive.
7. Control bleeding by firm pressure, not by clamps, in face injuries.

DISLOCATED SHOULDER

Immediately after a shoulder injury, tissue shock will enable you to manipulate the arm freely with little pain to the patient. Nevertheless, the less traumatic the method the better. One way is to let gravity do it for you by tying a 5-lb. weight to the patient's arm and letting it hang over the side of a table or cart.

If that's not possible, you can try gentle traction while externally rotating the arm; it helps to put your foot in the axilla (below), but use it as a fulcrum for the humerus to lever against rather than something to push with.

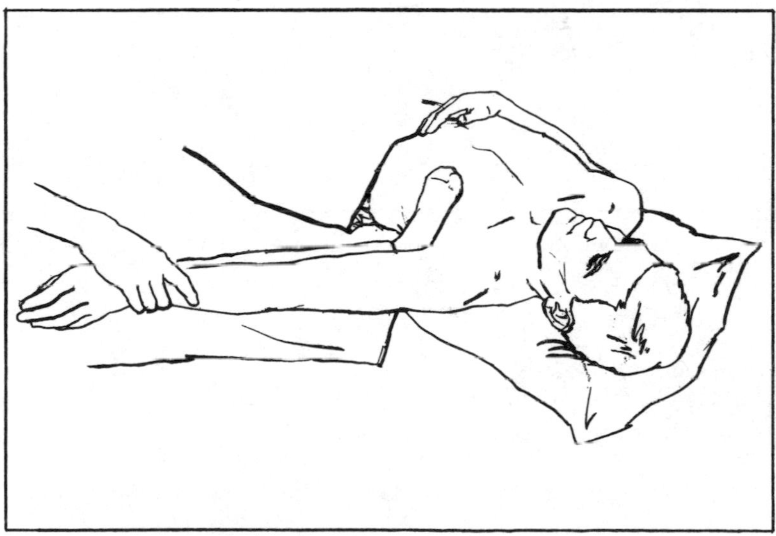

Figure 5. Dislocated Shoulder. Reprinted with permission from: *Emergency Medicine*. Copyright© by Merk & Co., Inc.

NOTES

Report and Record System

PROBLEMS—DATA—SOLUTIONS

REPORT SYSTEMS

A vital part of the SLS concept is that each patient will enter the Admitting area of the hospital with a simple, meaningful *record*. The record is to consist of *three lists* as follows:

I. Problems

List the **problems** the patient has had since you saw him. Obviously anything that bothers or is bad for the patient is a **problem. The problems should be listed in order of importance and assigned a code number.** For instance, **heart attack with cardiac arrest** will be assigned **#1 always.** As you will see later, in the section on Computerization in this manual, this will eventually allow you to push a button and receive instant instructions.

II. Data

The **data** list consists of the actual facts that you have available, facts that might be important for the next person who takes over to know. This list should include things that you learn from the family and patient and that you have observed yourself. For instance, the **data** regarding the heart attack victim mentioned above would include:

1. Chest pain for 2 months.
2. Took **digitalis**.
3. Took **nitroglycerin**.
4. Under care of Dr. Trogli.
5. Cardiac arrest on initial examination.
6. **Ventricular tachycardia** after external cardiac massage.
7. Normal sinus rhythm with **ventricular extra systoles** after 400 millisec of electric shock.
8. Normal sinus rhythm after 50 mg of **Lidocaine I.V.**

A fact can be both a **problem** and **data** and can be put in both lists. The **data** list will also eventually be assigned permanent numbers so that, when these code numbers are transmitted or designated, suggestions as to how they should be reacted to can be transmitted to you either via computer, dispatcher, or in a manual such as this.

III. Solutions

The **solutions** list should contain all that you have done to help the patient, again numbered consecutively at first and eventually by assigned code number. For instance, the heart patient **solutions** list would read:

Oxygen
Countershock—400 millisec × 3
Lidocaine—100 mg
I.V. Lactated Ringer's running

At this point you may realize that your **solutions** list may be a way by which you can check quality control in your team. *Certain* **problems** and *certain* **data** *should* lead to *certain* **solutions**; and when all of these are code numbered, a computer can check the matchups.

EXAMPLE OF A TYPICAL RECORD

NAME: John Doe Date: Time:
AGE: 42
BLOOD PRESSURE: 100/70—fill in last reading
PULSE: 60
PROBLEMS:
1. Chest pain
2. Heart stopped
3. Ventricular tachycardia

DATA:
1. History of heart trouble and chest pain
2. Taking heart pill once a day
3. Two brothers had heart attacks
4. EKG after external cardiac massage showed ventricular tachycardia (Patient now in normal sinus rhythm)

SOLUTIONS:
1. SLS Heart Arrest System
   External cardiac massage
   Bag breathing
   Oxygen
   Countershock—400 millisec × 3
   Lidocaine—100 mg I.V.
2. Lactated Ringer's with 500 mg of Lidocaine running

Signature: ______________________________

SLS Emergency Technician

Playlets to Demonstrate to the Community

SIMULATED LIFESAVING

PLAYLET DEMONSTRATIONS

Each SLS group should have a number of demonstration playlets to give to interested members of the community.

Acting out these playlets is, of course, an excellent teaching device. The more realistic they are, the more effective they are. We actually start the I.V.s and inject oranges while the playlets are being given.

Playlets are best developed from the day-to-day experiences of emergency personnel themselves.

SAMPLE PLAYLET DEMONSTRATIONS OF SLS

(When these are acted out with precision they act as a drill)

Playlet One

THE STRICKEN FOOTBALL COACH

A third string quarterback kicks a 72-yard field goal—his 38-year-old coach falls to the ground, not breathing. The SLS team standing on the sidelines arrives within seconds. Man #1 listens to the coach's heart, ascertaining it is **not** beating (note—he listens with a **stethoscope** and does not bother with the pulse). He starts **external cardiac massage**. Man #2 starts **bag breathing** (we think this more practicable than mouth-to-mouth) with O_2. Man #3 hooks patient up to the portable, battery powered EKG (a *sine qua non* of every emergency vehicle). As soon as he is hooked up he notes that the heart has started with **ventricular tachycardia** (a simple EKG pattern to read).

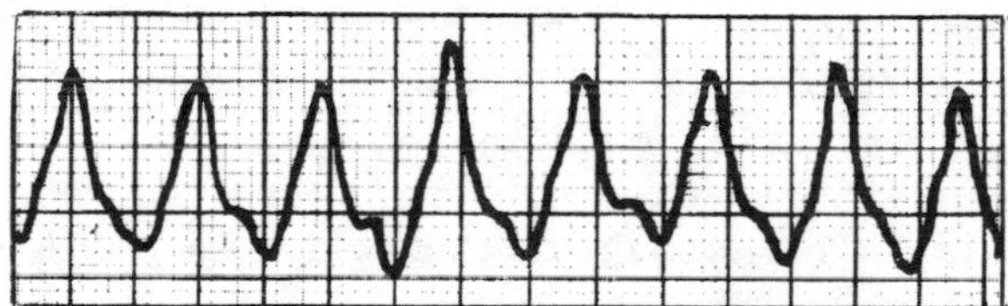

VENTRICULAR TACHYCARDIA

He informs the man doing the **massage** who stops and, as dictated by the System, gives 400 millisec of electric current. The rhythm stays the same. He gives another 400 millisec of current and the heart goes into **normal sinus rhythm** with **ventricular systole.**

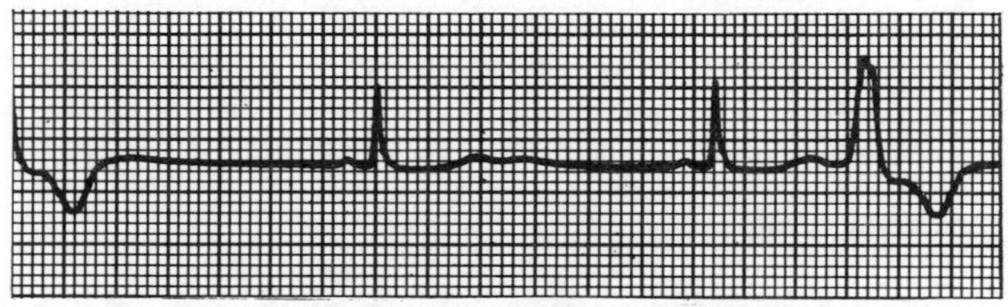

VENTRICULAR EXTRA SYSTOLE

The **bag** man keeps giving the O_2 although spontaneous breathing has started. (If a two-man team is here, a bystander can be the **bag man.**) Man #1 now starts an I.V. with Lactated Ringer's and injects a syringe full of **Lidocaine**, 100 mg (to stop the extra systoles) and he puts another syringe full of **Lidocaine**, 100 mg, into the bottle. He then injects an ampule of $NaHCO_3$ into the tubing (to prevent further arrhythmia).

While he is doing this man #3 is writing out the *report*:

PROBLEM:	Sudden collapse with heart stoppage.
DATA:	History of chest pain for 2 weeks—no previous medication—sequential EKG—**ventricular tachycardia—normal sinus rhythm** with **ventricular extra systole.**
SOLUTION:	**External cardiac massage—bag breathe O_2—electric shock × 2—Lidocaine,** 200 mg—I.V. $NaHCO_3$.

Man #2 now takes the blood pressure and finds it to be 110/70. If *below* 80 he would be prepared to put the **cardiogenic shock system** into effect—**Isuprel,** etc.

The patient arrives at the Admitting Ward intact. The EKG reports are given to the Admitting personnel.

The third string quarterback is hired right out of high school by the Philadelphia Eagles so the coach is ready to go back to work the next year.

Playlet Two
THE YOUNG DIABETIC IN A FREEWAY ACCIDENT

A 32-year-old diabetic is driving on the expressway. He loses consciousness. His car hits an abutment, pinning him, unconscious, inside. The steering wheel is broken, puncturing the right side of his chest.

The SLS Emergency Team arrives. Man #1 listens to the heart and states it is rapid and regular. Man #2 takes the blood pressure, which is 120/80. Man #3 starts an I.V. of Lactated Ringer's. Man #1 then pricks the patient's finger and does a **blood sugar**. Man #2 keeps the patient warm and bandages the chest wound, which is sucking air. The blood sugar is *less* than 20 and needle marks are noted on the man's thighs. Man #3 then puts 50 cc of 50% **glucose** in the I.V. and the patient regains consciouness. He complains of extreme difficulty in breathing and fullness in the chest. Man #3 makes a correct diagnosis of **tension pneumothorax** and places a #14 valve needle below the right clavicle, releasing the trapped air.

While the team is waiting for the welders to arrive to free the victim from the car, the **cardiac monitor** is placed and the **blood pressure** is taken *every* 15 minutes. Repeat finger prick is only 40, so another 50 cc of 50% **glucose** is given.

Report by #2 man:

PROBLEM:	Insulin coma
	Tension pneumothorax
	Shock
	Chest injury
DATA:	Blood sugar *less* than 30
	Severe pain in chest and feeling of "blowing up"
	Response to 50% **glucose**
	Blood pressure of 120/80
SOLUTIONS:	2 vials of 50% **glucose**
	#14 valve needle for tension pneumothorax
	2 liters of Lactated Ringer's
	Warmth for shock
	Compression dressing for chest wound

NOTES

Contests Between Simulated Lifesaving Teams

Groups that have mastered this manual should challenge others who are engaged in emergency care. The following modus operandi is suggested and in the fine American tradition of competition, groups can compare and improve their skills to their own and the patients' benefits.

SIMULATED LIFESAVING CONTESTS

After our initial course in Simulated Lifesaving, we felt a natural urge to compete with other groups, using the knowledge we had gained. We therefore proposed a National SLS Contest and issued a challenge. So few contestants appeared that we decided to push back the date of the National Contest to June, 1974.

One of the main stimuli to the writing of the Manual is the wish to make available to interested emergency personnel the type of material necessary for the training of a Simulated Lifesaving Team.

Competition is, of course, a great motivational force in learning. We hope that contests of the kind proposed will spring up to help everybody to thoroughly grasp the knowledge necessary for them to be really helpful to their neighbors in an emergency.

DIRECTIONS FOR SLS CONTEST

Each team of three men is given the **problem**. They have 3 minutes to digest it and plan their course of action.

A **patient** is supplied. He had either agreed to have an I.V. with Lactated Ringer's started on him or this will be simulated.

Each team uses its own **Jump Kit**. They are to actually take EKGs but the judge will hand them an EKG strip to interpret.

Beginning Teams may use ping pong paddles to simulate the electrical converter.

The two playlet problems will be used as examples.

Each judge will have a check sheet on which he builds up the Teams' total points.

PROBLEM

PROBLEM: A third string quarterback kicks a 72-yard field goal—his 38-year-old coach falls unconscious to the ground. An SLS team of three men is standing by.

JUDGING SEQUENCE

	No. of Points	Record No. if Given
1. Order of Examination: First action—listening to heart with stethoscope. As soon as you see him listening, tell him there are **no** heart sounds.	20	20
2. Starts **external cardiac massage**		
technique	20	10
Rhythm (45–60/minute)	20	20
3. Starts **bag breathing**:		
Checks **airway**	10	10
Technique	20	15
Rate 10–14	10	10
4. EKG hookup and quality of reading	30	
Give team EKG strip showing ventricular tachycardia		
a. External massage **stopped**	10	10
Tell them breathing has started		
b. **Bag breathing stopped but oxygen continued**	20	10
5. **Technique of electrical stimulation**		
a. Facility in setting up machine	80	50
b. Technique of **shocking**	80	
Tell them shock not successful		
c. Repeat **shock** (shock #2)	50	50
Repeat this three times—They get 50 for each repeat (shocks #2, #3, and #4)	150	150
On fourth shock tell them they have converted and give them EKG strip with NSR with **ventricular extra systoles**	50	50

		No. of Points	Record No. if Given
6.	I.V. with Lactated Ringer's—technique with I.V.	100	50
7.	Injection of bolus of Lidocaine	100	50
8.	Injection of 50 mg of Lidocaine into I.V.	100	50
9.	**Report**		
	Problem:Heart stopped	25	25
	Ventricular tachycardia	25	25
	Ventricular extra systoles	25	—
	Date: EKG showed ventricular tachy-cardia then NSR with ventricular	25	25
	extra systoles	25	25
	Blood pressure 120/70	50	50
	Solution: Cardiac massage	50	50
	Bag breathing	50	50
	Five electrical **shocks** at 400 mEq/sec	50	50
	50 mg Lidocaine by bolus	50	—
	50 mg Lidocaine in I.V. running	50	—
Ready to transport:			
	Blood pressure cuff on	50	50
	O_2 running	50	—
	Patient sitting in upright position	50	25
	Monitor going	50	—
		1495	930

The above hypothetical team then scored 930 out of a possible 1495.

DIRECTIONS FOR JUDGING THE "DIABETIC ON THE FREEWAY ACCIDENT" PROBLEM

PROBLEM: (Note—the victim is given a neck tag on which is printed "I am a **diabetic.**")

A 32-year-old man is found unconscious in his wrecked car along a freeway abutment. The steering wheel has punctured his right chest. (Pinned to the victim's shirt is a patch labelled "Puncture wound from steering wheel.") A three-man SLS team arrives.

JUDGING SEQUENCE	POINTS	GIVEN
1. **SLS man #1** listens to chest with a stethoscope. He is told heart is regular at 110.	50	50
2. **SLS man #2** checks airway. He is told it is open and respirations are 14.	25	—
3. **SLS man #3** takes the blood pressure. He is told it is 130/70.	50	50
4. **SLS man #1**, being told that airway, heart, and blood pressure are okay, does a finger prick blood sugar. It is less than 30.	50	50
5. An I.V. with Lactated Ringer's is then started and into the tubing is put 100 cc of 50% glucose. The patient is instructed to wake up, but then lapses into coma again.	100	75
6. He is given another 100 cc of 50% glucose.	50	50

	POINTS	GIVEN
7. When the victim awakens he starts complaining of difficulty in breathing and a feeling of "blowing up" inside. (The team is informed that the wound has begun to suck air on inspiration.) The SLS team then places a #14 valve needle below the clavicle (simulated, of course) to release the air and puts a sterile, air tight dressing over the chest wound.	100	—
	425	275

They cover him with a blanket and inform the judge the patient is ready for transport.

The team has earned 275 points out of a possible 425. Points are given not only for simulated procedures but for the techniques of their performance.

NOTES

Practical Aids

PROFICIENCY CARD

CHECK SHEET FOR CERTIFICATE OF UNDERSTANDING OF THE VARIOUS ELEMENTS OF THE SIMULATED LIFESAVING SYSTEM

SOME THOUGHTS FOR THE PHYSICIAN-DIRECTORS AND TEACHERS OF THE SLS COURSES

COMPUTERIZATION OF THE MANUAL

THE "DREAM"

EKG FLASH CARDS

PROFICIENCY CARD

Rather than a formal diploma for a SLS Course the following **Proficiency Card** is suggested after the check sheet that follows has had each element initialled by the Directing Physician. The signature of the appropriate Directing Physician on the **Proficiency Card** signifies that the individual has satisfied the Directing Physician, regarding his proficiency in a procedure, well enough for the physician to be willing to direct the individual to use the procedure in an emergency (if it is possible in his area) on a patient for whom the physician has the primary reponsibility.

---

has demonstrated to my satisfaction that he understands and can use the following emergency procedures and systems well enough that I would direct him to use them on my patients in an emergency.

Signature **Date**

Cardiac Resuscitation—Cardiologist
Endotracheal Intubation—Anesthesiologist
Ob/Gyn—Obstetrician-Gynecologist

The Table of Contents of this manual can then be appended.

Check Sheet For
CERTIFICATE OF UNDERSTANDING OF THE VARIOUS ELEMENTS OF THE SIMULATED LIFESAVING SYSTEM

Each SLS graduate is checked out on his understanding, in simulated problems, and actual use of each element of this Jump Kit and of the recommended drugs carried in the ambulance; his recognition of the most important EKGs; and his understanding of the **Systems** for differing situations. The Directing Physician will indicate that the SLS graduate has demonstrated his understanding of an element by initialling it.

	DATE	INITIAL
Stethoscope		
Blood Pressure Cuff		
Bag Mask Respirator with O_2 Hookup		
Airway Kit—Suction Machine, Pharyngeal Airway, McGill Forceps, Laryngoscope and Endotracheal Tube, Emergency Tracheostomy Needle, Esophageal Airway		
Heimlich Maneuver		
Four Tourniquets		
First Aid Kit		
Spine Board		
Intravenous Set with Stand and Instructions for Use		
Disposable Sterile Stylets for Finger Pricks		
Blood Sugar Finger Prick Sticks		
#14 Gage Needle with Valve for Tension Pneumothorax		
Urinary Catheter Set		
Defibrillator with Heart Monitor—Both Visual and Readout		

The Directing Physician initials the SLS graduate's understanding of each **drug:**

	DATE	INITIAL
Adrenalin		
Aminophyllin		
Amytal		
Atropine		
Compazine		
Demerol		
Dextrose (50% Glucose)		
Diazoxide		
Digoxin		
Dopamine		
Ergotrate		
Insulin		
Lasix		
Narcan		
Nitroglycerin		
Propranolol		
Reactose Tablets		
Ringer's Lactate		
Sodabicarb		
Solu-Cortef		
Valium		
Xylocaine		

The Directing Physician also confirms, with his initials, the SLS graduate's ability to recognize the most important EKG patterns.

	DATE	INITIAL
Normal Sinus Rhythm		
Ventricular Extra Systoles		
Ventricular Tachycardia		
Ventricular Fibrillation		
Sinus Bradycardia		

The Directing Physician also affirms, with his initials, the SLS graduate's understanding of the various Systems.

	DATE	INITIAL
Resuscitation, with normal sinus rhythm after cardiac arrest		
Resuscitation, with normal sinus rhythm with ventricular extra systoles after cardiac arrest		
Resuscitation, with ventricular tachycardia after cardiac arrest		
Resuscitation, with ventricular fibrillation after cardiac arrest		
Resuscitation, with sinus bradycardia after cardiac arrest		
System for the unconscious patient		
System for diabetic coma		
System for heart attack		
System for congestive heart failure		
System for shock		
System for stroke or brain hemorrhage		
System for drug overdose		
System for auto accident injuries		
System for chest injury		
System for gastrointestinal tract bleeding		
System for woman in labor or bleeding from the vagina		
System for burn management		
System for lung failure		
System for carbon monoxide poisoning		
System for emergency care of the eyes		
System for insulin reaction		
System for allergic reaction		
System for drowning		
System for initial care of spine injury		
System for severe head injury		

SOME THOUGHTS FOR THE PHYSICIAN-DIRECTORS AND TEACHERS OF SLS COURSES

If you have been actively engaged in the care of severely ill patients I think most of what is in this manual will be perfectly understandable to you. If your experience has been administrative or strictly academic, this manual is **not** for you.

You might be interested in some principles that have occurred to me as I have tried to teach emergency personnel.

First, these men are fundamentally activists. If they had been traditional students their natural intelligence (which is impressive to me) would have directed them into other fields. Therefore, traditional lectures will not get points across to them. Each session should be carefully planned as to content, but when interest wanes in a segment it should be quickly changed. At each session work on understanding the "jump kit," techniques, and specific System development.

During most of the 90-minute sessions everyone should be standing.

A total of fifteen men at each session seems all that is practicable.

Each System should be built up by the group itself, with the instructor incorporating his own ideas and prejudices, so the final System for your particular group is typed in on the blank pages that follow the Systems worked out by my test groups.

The more **doing** the men perform each session, the more **learning** seems to take place. Therefore, always start out with a specific problem and work from there.

Skills, such as starting I.V.s, giving intramuscular injections, and reading EKGs need to be practiced over and over. We find starting I.V.s, doing finger prick blood sugars, and taking EKGs can best be done on each other. Intramuscular injections are best practiced on oranges. Intratracheal intubation and childbirth care are best done on mannequins.

How the men will eventually be able to put this knowledge to work will be essentially a local problem, which will be loaded with political overtones. However, I feel that there must be large groups of practicing physicians, such as myself, who want their patients to be better cared for in an emergency situation and who are willing to teach emergency personnel what to do. If you number yourself among these you will enjoy teaching these men, who are dedicated indeed. I do not see how the knowledge we impart can be prevented from eventually helping our patients.

Finally, involve as many of your colleagues as possible in teaching the emergency personnel. The men can benefit from many points of view and I have found that, when physicians become involved in teaching SLS, they become convinced that it has a place in the general scheme of total patient care.

Remember, physicians have become accustomed to a highly technical language of their own. Tell your audience to interrupt you every time you use a word they do not understand. If they do this, you will soon get in the habit of simplifying your language. The definitions at the back of this manual may be of some help in this regard.

COMPUTERIZATION OF THE MANUAL*

This manual has been written for eventual computerization and this can be accomplished with a teletype terminal that can be hooked into a portable telephone. The actual computer storage can be on any large time-sharing computer that may be leased in your area.

The System will eventually tie in with an inevitable area-wide Medical Record System, in which a person's Social Security number will act as the ingress to his pertinent medical record.

The programming of the Manual is a straightforward programming problem for an expert but, should a community want the program for immediate use, it is available commercially.*

The following hypothetical example illustrates how this would work.

1. John Doe, Soc. Sec. #123-45-6789, has a heart attack and you arrive.
2. You hook your portable computer terminal to your telephone and type 123-45-6789. This will go to his medical record.
3. Your teletype replies: Name-John Doe. Heart attack-1968. On **Coumadin** and **Digitalis**. What has happened?
4. You type: Severe chest pain. EKG—normal sinus rhythm with ventricular extra systoles.
5. Teletype replies with a reproduction of page 86—the **Heart Attack System.**

What your community and its physicians decide in regard to how far you and the computer can go is conjectural, but you **can** see, even at this point, that modern applications are there for the taking—and at small expense—since computer terminals and time are all available on lease in every large community.

*Get in touch with the author of the Manual.

THE DREAM

The **Dream** is that among every large group of Americans there would be several who had mastered the contents of this Manual and who would have the authorization from a physician to put their knowledge into play.

In each large building a "jump kit" would be available and kept up-to-date, similar to the way a fire extinguisher is now available on each floor of such a building.

When someone had a heart attack in that building, an alarm would ring and the qualified personnel would arrive within minutes to start the "heart attack" program.

Training in **simulated lifesaving** would start in high school (several high school students were in our pilot course). With strategically placed "jump kits" and universal SLS training, Americans would be able to help each other in many situations, where now they stand powerless at the scene of a catastrophe.

NOTES

A SELF-TEACH COURSE IN EKGs

Cut EKGs along dotted lines.

Learn to recognize and pick out of the resulting flash cards the five that represent ventricular rhythms—within 20 seconds. These are the arrhythmias you will react to in the ambulance situation. *Ignore* the other rhythms.

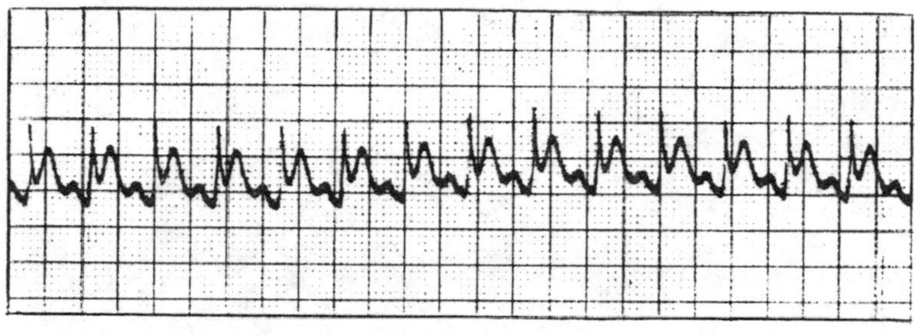

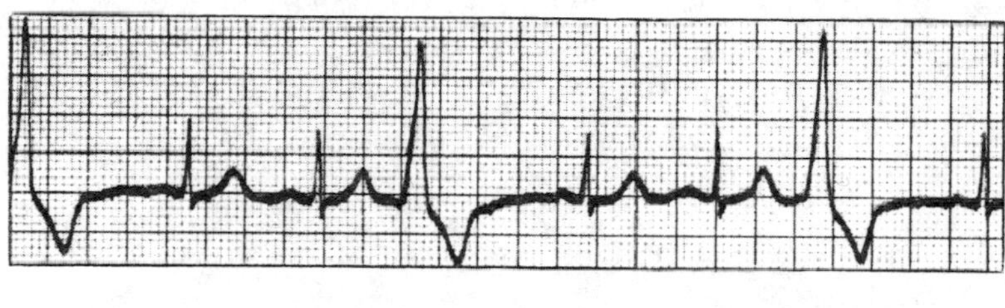

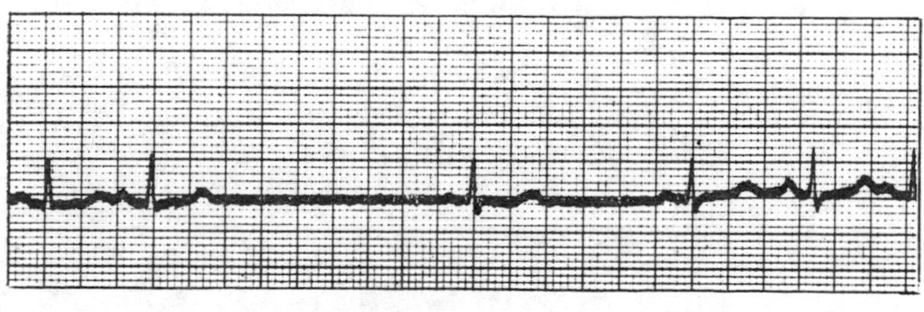

(PAROXYSMAL) ATRIAL TACHYCARDIA

FREQUENT PREMATURE VENTRICULAR CONTRACTIONS

SINUS ARREST

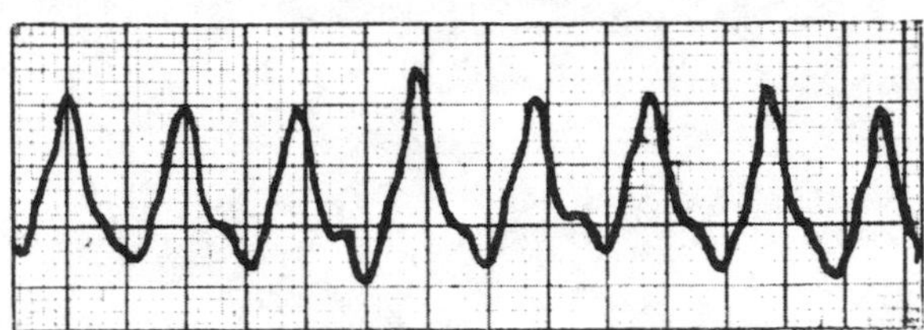

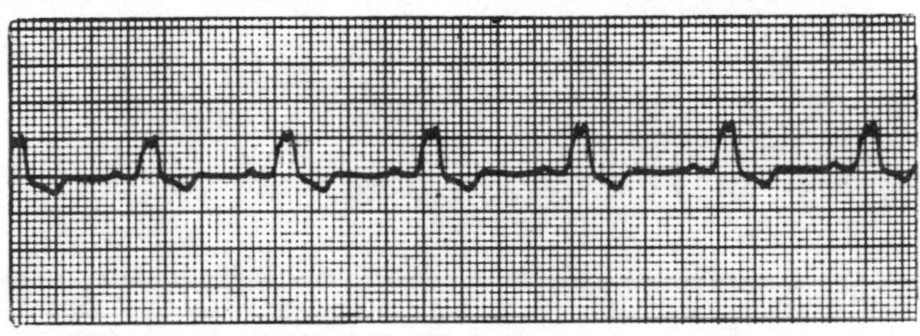

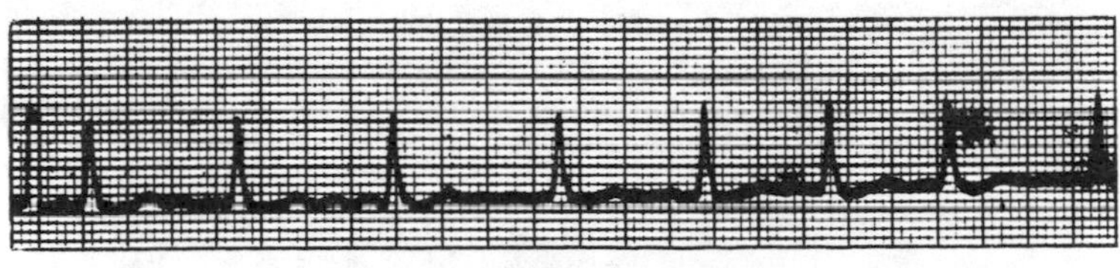

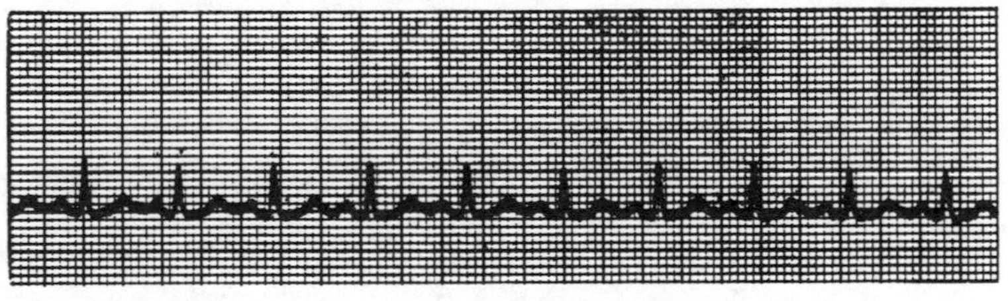

VENTRICULAR TACHYCARDIA

LEFT BUNDLE BRANCH BLOCK

ATRIAL FIBRILLATION

SINUS TACHYCARDIA

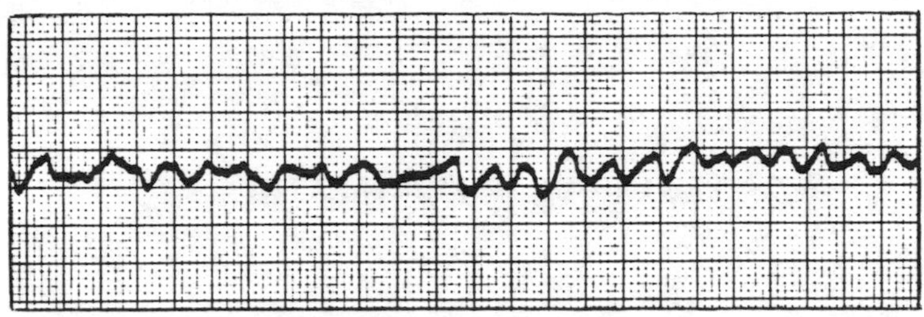

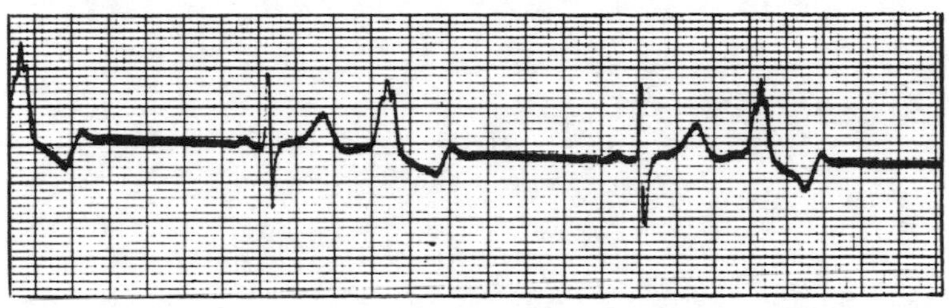

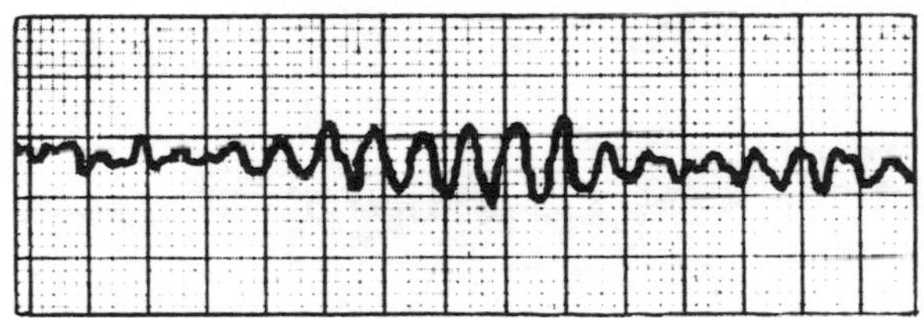

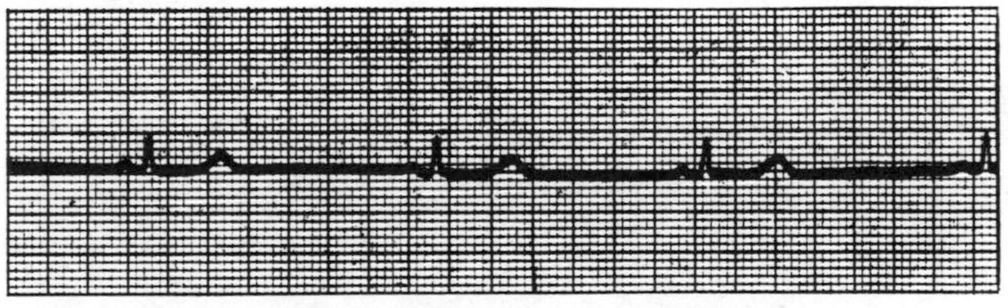

VENTRICULAR FIBRILLATION

FREQUENT PVCs PRODUCING BIGEMINY

VENTRICULAR FIBRILLATION

SINUS BRADYCARDIA

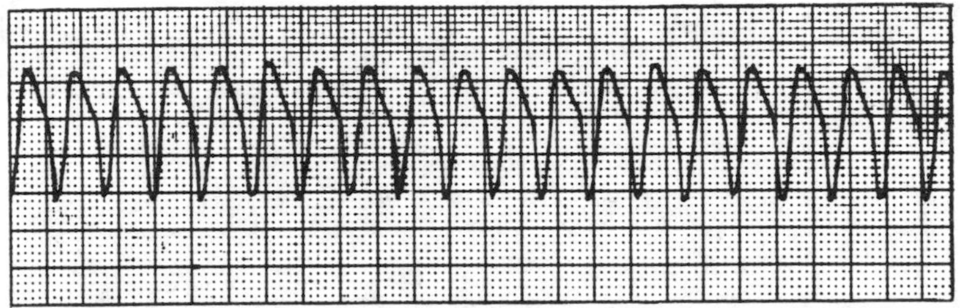

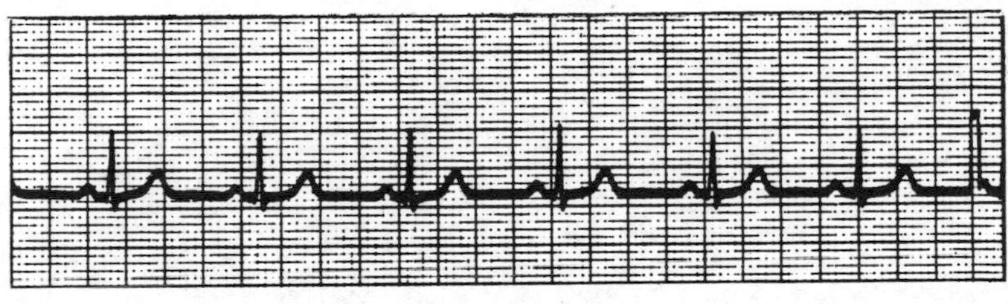

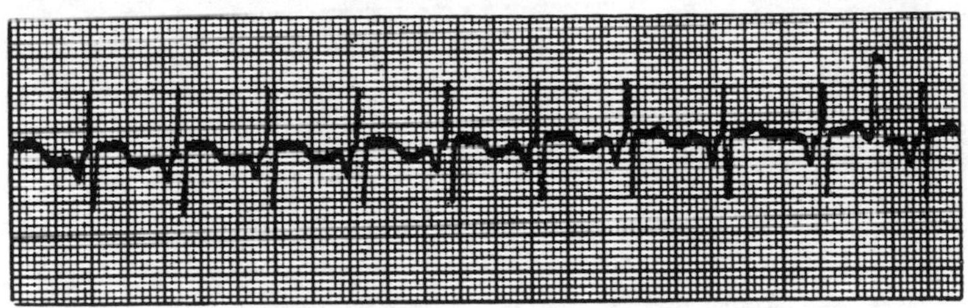

VENTRICULAR TACHYCARDIA

NORMAL SINUS

NODAL TACHYCARDIA

Definitions of Words

DEFINITIONS OF WORDS

Adrenal Glands — Glands located just above the kidneys. They secrete adrenalin and cortisone into the blood stream.

Antagonist — Used to describe drugs that inactivate drugs such as Nalline and Morphine.

Anaphylaxis — An acute allergic reaction that often is fatal. It can and should be treated with Adrenalin.

Arrhythmia — Describes situation when heart is not beating either at normal rate or regularly.

Asthma — Asthma is a disease in which the patient wheezes because he cannot get air out of his lungs as the outflow passages have been partially closed by a spasm due to an allergy. In extreme cases the patient can die from lack of oxygen. Adrenalin is used to relieve the spasm.

Auricle — The filling chambers of the heart, from which heart beats are supposed to originate.

Bag Mask — A rubber mask to go over the nose and mouth. It is attached to a rubber canister, which is compressed by hand to drive air into the lungs, then expands to fill with air again.

Barbiturate	A class of drug that acts as a depressant. So-called "downers" include seconal, nembutal, tuinal, and phenobarbital. Treatment of overdose is attention to breathing and I.V. Lactated Ringer's.
Blood Sugar	The amount of glucose or sugar in the blood—70 mg/ml is lower limit of normal, 120 mg/ml is upper limit of normal.
Bronchus	Either one of two main branches of trachea.
Cardiac Arrest	The heart has stopped beating.
Cardiologist	A physician who specializes in treating heart disease.
Coma	This is another name for unconsciousness.
Diabetic Coma	Unconsciousness due to uncontrolled diabetes and serious lack of insulin.
Directing Physicians	In this Manual this refers to the physicians in your community who are willing to take responsibility for decision making, both in regard to directing you (**within the limits of the law**) to do things that might help their patients. Directing Physicians are the key men in the SLS concept and I assume the busiest ambulance drivers will be able to determine who are the best and busiest physicians in their community to approach for this vital function.

Defibrillator A machine that will apply direct current to the chest wall through two paddles—to start the heart or convert it to an acceptable rhythm.

Diluent A substance used to dissolve a drug that comes in powder form.

Diuretic A drug given to provoke urine output.

Electrocardiogram The strip of special paper on which the electrical action of the heart is recorded.

EKG An electrocardiogram, that is, an electrical picture of the heart action.

Electrical Defibrillation A device designed to deliver electric shock to the heart in order to change the rhythm of the heart—or in some cases to start it.

Endotracheal Tube A soft tube that goes into the trachea to provide direct access of oxygen into the lungs.

Epiglottis A fibrous valve that closes off the bronchus during swallowing and opens during breathing.

External Cardiac Massage Pressure, by the heels of the hands, on the front of the chest to force blood in and out of a heart that is not beating. Readers of this Manual should be familiar with this technique from their Emergency Technician courses.

Heart Attack	Blockage of a blood vessel that supplies the wall of the ventricle of the heart and causes pain—sometimes shock—sometimes heart irregularites.
Hyperglycemia	Too much sugar in the blood—usually diabetes. Treatment is insulin.
Hypoglycemia	Too little sugar in the blood—treatment is 50% glucose.
I.M.	Intramuscularly—by a needle into the muscle.
Intravenous	Into the vein.
I.V.	Intravenous or intravenously—that is, by means of a needle introduced into the vein.
Jump Kit	A slang expression used in this Manual to describe the equipment brought to the scene of the accident by the ambulance. It derives its name from the ambulance medics.
Laryngoscope	An instrument with a light on the end that is placed through the mouth to enable you to see the vocal cords so that you can get a tube into the bronchi.
Lidocaine	A drug that acts to "freeze" the heart muscle so that it does not react to stimuli (which ordinarily would make it beat) from an abnormal focus in the ventricle, which was caused by acute heart damage.

Mannequin	A plastic model of the human body, used to practice cardiopulmonary resuscitation and the insertion of endotracheal tubes.
McGill Forceps	A long, curved forceps that can be used to extract chunks of food or tissue out of the back of the throat or pharynx.
mg	Milligram, the unit of weight many drugs are prescribed in.
Oscilloscope	A device that shows the EKG pattern on a screen or large bulb.
Pharynx	Back portion of the throat.
Pharyngeal	The part of the throat between the mouth and the trachea and esophagus.
Ringer's (Lactated)	Lactated Ringer's is the common name for the intravenous fluid used in this Manual.
Shock	A condition of low blood pressure caused by inadequate oxygen being brought to the body cells by the blood stream.
Simulated Lifesaving	A pretend type of lifesaving in which all training and practice is done on well persons with their permission.
S.Q.	Subcutaneously—by a needle placed under the skin but not into the muscle.

Suction Machine A machine that creates negative pressure so that a tube attached to it will be able to pull out foreign obstructions and secretions from the throat or an endotracheal tube.

System A system is an orderly way of accomplishing a goal—doing it the same way each time.

Systems Method A systems method is a way of doing something by first breaking the entire action into its component parts and then building up the procedure by attending to those component parts in orderly fashion.

NOTES

Index

INDEX